Seeing Through New Eyes

of related interest

Understanding Sensory Dysfunction
Learning, Development and Sensory Dysfunction in Autism Spectrum Disorders,
ADHD, Learning Disabilities and Bipolar Disorder
Polly Godwin Emmons and Liz McKendry Anderson
ISBN-13: 978 1 84310 806 1   ISBN-10: 1 84310 806 2

Sensory Perceptual Issues in Autism and Asperger Syndrome
Different Sensory Experiences – Different Perceptual Worlds
Olga Bogdashina
Forewords by Wendy Lawson and Theo Peeters
ISBN-13: 978 1 84310 166 6   ISBN-10: 1 84310 166 1

Sensory Smarts
A Book for Kids with ADHD or Autism Spectrum Disorders Struggling with
Sensory Integration Problems
Kathleen A. Chara and Paul J. Chara, Jr. with Christian P. Chara
Illustrated by J.M. Berns
ISBN-13: 978 1 84310 783 5   ISBN-10: 1 84310 783 X

Asperger's Syndrome
A Guide for Parents and Professionals
Tony Attwood
Foreword by Lorna Wing
ISBN-13: 978 1 85302 577 8   ISBN-10: 1 85302 577 1

Assessing and Developing Communication and Thinking Skills in People
with Autism and Communication Difficulties
A Toolkit for Parents and Professionals
Kate Silver, Autism Initiatives
ISBN-13: 978 1 84310 352 3   ISBN-10: 1 84310 352 4

Pre-Schoolers with Autism
An Education and Skills Training Programme for Parents
Manual for Clinicians and Manual for Parents
Avril V. Brereton and Bruce J. Tonge
Manual for Clinicians ISBN-13: 978 1 84310 341 7   ISBN-10: 1 84310 341 9
Manual for Parents ISBN-13: 978 1 84310 342 4   ISBN-10: 1 84310 342 7

Seeing Through New Eyes

Changing the Lives of Children with Autism, Asperger Syndrome and Other Developmental Disabilities Through Vision Therapy

Melvin Kaplan

Foreword by Stephen M. Edelson

Jessica Kingsley Publishers
London and Philadelphia

First published in 2006
by Jessica Kingsley Publishers
116 Pentonville Road
London N1 9JB, UK
and
400 Market Street, Suite 400
Philadelphia, PA 19106, USA

www.jkp.com

The Appendix originally appeared as "The Van Orden Star: A window into personal space" in the *Journal of Optometric Vision Development 33*, 1, 21–28 (2002). Reproduced by kind permission of the College of Optometrists in Vision Development.

Library of Congress Cataloging in Publication Data
Kaplan, Melvin, 1929-
  Seeing through new eyes : changing the lives of children with autism, Asperger syndrome and other developmental disabilities through vision therapy / Melvin Kaplan ; foreword by Stephen Edelson.— 1st American pbk. ed.
    p. cm.
Includes index.
  ISBN-13: 978-1-84310-800-9 (pbk. : alk. paper)
  ISBN-10: 1-84310-800-3 (pbk. : alk. paper) 1. Asperger's syndrome. 2. Autism. 3. Autism in children.
    [DNLM: 1. Vision Disorders—complications—Child—Case Reports. 2. Vision Disorders—therapy—Child—Case Reports. 3. Autistic Disorder—complications—Child—Case Reports. 4. Developmental Disabilities—complications—Child—Case Reports. WW 600 K17s 2006]
I. Title.
  RC553.A88.K37 2006
  616.85'88—dc22

2005023412

British Library Cataloguing in Publication Data
A CIP catalogue record for this book is available from the British Library

ISBN-13: 978 1 84310 800 9
ISBN-10: 1 84310 800 3

Printed and Bound in the United States by Thomson-Shore, Inc.

Contents

For their love, support, and patience – my wife Ellen, and my children Marla, Stuart, David, and the memory of Jeffrey.

Foreword

Doctors treating autism and other developmental disabilities often give parents a bleak picture of their children's future. These disorders, they typically say, are untreatable except with psychotropic drugs that mask behavioral symptoms without correcting core problems.

Fortunately, these doctors are wrong. In reality, mounting evidence clearly shows that autism and related developmental disabilities are very much treatable. A wide range of therapies—among them intensive one-on-one educational intervention, special diets, nutritional therapies, and sensory integration therapy—are dramatically changing the lives of hundreds of thousands of children once considered "hopeless."

How does vision fit into this picture? The visual system is our dominant sense—more information is obtained by the visual sensory system than by any other sensory system. As Dr. Kaplan explains in this book, a remarkably high percentage of children with autism and other developmental and cognitive problems suffer from vision problems that severely impair their attention, their ability to understand their world, and their ability to respond to the people around them. Dr. Kaplan and his colleagues (including myself) have published research demonstrating that visual training frequently can successfully address these vision problems, and in the process allow children to open up to a world once closed to them. Vision therapy works synergistically with other interventions, enabling children to respond much more positively to educational interventions and other sensory integration therapies.

I first met Dr. Kaplan in the mid-1990s, at a time when his autistic patient load was increasing exponentially due to "word of mouth" in the autism community. After hearing many positive reports from parents who brought their autistic children to see him, I was anxious to find out more about his work. Because my graduate training was in experimental psychology, I was initially dubious about the relationship of visual dysfunction to the problems of children with autism or other developmental disabilities. However, while I typically am a bit skeptical of a new treatment at first, I am, at the same time, always excited about the possibility of another potentially effective treatment option.

After watching Dr. Kaplan's lecture at a conference and then grilling him afterwards about the reasoning behind the treatment, I soon realized the key role that vision therapy can play in treating many individuals with autism and related disabilities. Over the years, I have had the opportunity to watch Dr. Kaplan work with many patients in his clinic in Tarrytown, New York as well as in Canada and Italy, and I've been amazed at how the yoked prism lenses he uses can have an immediate impact on a child's behavior and response to the environment. I have seen remarkable changes in these children and adults right before my eyes. Some of the memorable improvements include:

- an immediate change from toe-walking to normal, flat walking

- much better hand–eye coordination

- better posture in sitting and walking

- a change from hyperactive and inattentive behavior to calm and attentive behavior.

These instant changes can translate, with the help of vision therapy, into long-term changes including better attention, increased speech, enhanced social skills, and better academic performance. They also can result in a happier, less anxious, less tense individual, with more energy to understand and enjoy the world.

In addition to his contributions as a dedicated clinician, Dr. Kaplan deserves recognition as a true pioneer in the field of vision training. One of the most notable aspects of his work is that he made many of his first ground-breaking discoveries about the role of vision problems in developmental and psychiatric disorders in the 1970s—an era in which most professionals were still uniformly blaming many such disorders on poor parenting or early emotional trauma. Dr. Kaplan's use of vision therapy to help patients with schizophrenia and anxiety disorders in the late 1970s and early 1980s, an approach that flew in the face of medical dogma, made him one of the first medical professionals to offer an effective biological treatment for these patients. He continues, to this day, to challenge the medical establishment—and he continues to persevere in seeking the most effective ways to improve the lives of the children and adults he treats.

Stephen M. Edelson, Ph.D.
Autism Research Institute
San Diego, CA

Part I

Understanding Visual Dysfunction and the Role of Prism Lenses and Vision Therapy

CHAPTER 1

The Behavior is the Solution

We don't think of autism spectrum disorders, hyperactivity, and other learning and behavior disorders as problems that involve visual dysfunction, but we should. That's because vision involves the brain as well as the eyes, and many disabled children suffer from neurological problems that prevent them from correctly perceiving what their eyes see. These perceptual deficits can translate into impaired social skills, poor language skills, motor problems, and a host of other severe symptoms—even in children with 20/20 eyesight.

Why do vision problems have such far-reaching consequences? The human organism is a "spatial action system," and most of the information we receive from our environment comes from our visual processes. When these processes break down, the result can be catastrophic—because seeing a world that's distorted, fragmented, two-dimensional, or incomprehensible can be as disabling as not seeing anything at all.

Frequently, disabled children or adults respond to the confusion and fear created by visual impairment by developing the symptoms that doctors see as "problems"—rocking, hand-flapping, toe-walking, poor eye contact, social withdrawal, tantrums, odd posture, rituals, hyperactivity. If you are a clinician, the most important idea I will ask you to consider in this book is to see these symptoms not as problems, but as *solutions* to problems. By viewing the behaviors of your patients as clues, and allowing these clues to guide you to the correct treatments for your patients' visual deficits, you will discover that you can free these individuals to see their once-frightening world in a new and exciting way.

> Anna, a nonverbal autistic eight-year-old, failed to respond to puzzles, the TV, a game of catch, or any other activities until I placed a pair of ambient prism lenses on her face. Instantly, she rose and began exploring the room, stopping in front of a full-length mirror to dance.
>
> When I attempted to remove the lenses, she held them tightly to her face and cried, "My eyes! My eyes!"

I'm not a fan of labels in my practice. The patients I see have lots of these labels—autistic, learning disabled, emotionally disturbed, hyperactive, attention disordered—but I don't view people with disabilities as different. Instead, I view them as having different levels of visual performance.

Visual performance can be conceived as a bell curve, with optimal performance at the peak. On one end of the curve are people who experience visual *compression*, and at the other end are those who experience visual *disparity*. I'll discuss both of these perceptual problems later, but for now it's important simply to understand that almost nobody is at the peak of this bell curve. To some degree, we are all autistic, or learning disabled, or attention disordered, because our vision doesn't work perfectly.

For most of us, however, this visual dysfunction is mild enough to masquerade as normal behavior or slight eccentricity. For instance, you might know a person who says, "Don't talk to me while I'm driving." Or maybe you know someone who can't tell left from right, or reads with one eye shut. All of these are ways of coping with visual dysfunction.

What is the difference between these people, and Anna, my nonverbal autistic patient? It's simply a matter of degree: the greater the degree of sensory dysfunction, the harder it becomes to process information, and to organize and orient to the environment—and, as a result, the harder it is to behave in what we consider a "normal" way.

The brain can be compared to a system of roads, with information traveling from one location to another. If the roads are direct and smooth, travel is easy. If construction creates a barrier, however, the highway is blocked and traffic may be redirected into clogged side streets. There is still movement, but it is slow and frustrating. Children with severe visual dysfunction spend too much time on these side streets, and the simple act of perceiving the world, and reacting to that perception, becomes a nightmare.

From vision problems to behavior problems

The children I treat have varying levels of visual problems, and the more severe their problems, the more pronounced the behavioral and academic effects. Here is a hierarchy of the effects of increasingly severe visual dysfunction:

Level 1:   Problems with reading; difficulty with physical activity and sports; some types of social problems.

Level 2:   Problems with visual organization and depth perception. This can manifest as anxiety, panic, or difficulty with night vision.

Level 3:   Weakness in visual organization and visual orientation. This severe level of visual dysfunction can contribute to autistic behavior, as well as to symptoms of bipolar disorder and schizophrenia.

Of course, children with behavioral problems have multiple sensory issues, and visual dysfunction is just one of them. But because 80 percent of the information we receive from our environment is visual, the visual aspect of sensory dysfunction can have far-reaching and devastating consequences. It is hard to overestimate the difficulty of functioning in a world where you can't tell where you are, where other people are, where objects are, or even where your body ends and the outside world begins.

To show a parent or professional just how debilitating visual dysfunction can be, I like to offer a real-life example. To do this, I set up two chairs, 10 to 15 feet apart, and ask my subject to sit in one of the chairs. Then I ask the person to stand up, walk to the other chair, and sit down on it without "feeling" for it by hand. It's a simple task, and no one has any trouble performing it.

Next, I place disruptive ambient lenses on my subject, and ask, "Can you see the other chair?" The answer is always "Yes," because ambient lenses have no effect on the ability to identify an object. I then ask my subject, once again, to walk to the other chair.

When people try this with the disruptive lenses in the "down" position, they knock over the chair. When they try it with the lenses in the "up" position, they stop short of the chair. Their loss of orientation affects their vestibular system, and they feel as if the room is swaying. Fearful, they respond by slowing down, shifting their bodies forward or back, toe-walking, or waving their arms as they walk. All of these are consistent with the "stims" we see in autism.

The people who participate in this experiment move from an ordered view to a disordered view, and within minutes they develop "symptoms" as a result. I ask them to imagine what it's like to live in that disordered world not for a few minutes, but for a lifetime.

Another way in which I help parents and professionals comprehend the disabling effects of visual dysfunction is to correct their own (usually relatively mild) visual deficits. One day, for instance, while I was working with the five-year-old daughter of an attorney named Jim, he asked me, "Why does she respond so well to the lenses?" Rather than simply telling him, I showed him.

First, I conducted a few quick tests that allowed me to identify Jim's perceptual style. Then I asked him, "Did you ever play sports?" He said yes—he'd played football, as a linebacker. "Your perceptual style tells me that you'd defend well in the outside, but you'd have trouble over the middle," I told him. "Let me show you why."

I threw a ball to him, and although he caught it, his timing was off and he caught it close to his body. Then I gave him ambient lenses, and threw the ball to him again. This time, he reached out and caught it easily. Shaking his head, he said, "I could have been a pro." He shared that he'd played on a university team, but his timing was off and he wasn't picked by the professional scouts.

Jim's subtle visual impairment cost him a chance at a professional sports career, but it didn't seriously affect his ability to function in other areas. The patients I typically see, however—patients like Jim's daughter—are much further from optimal on the bell curve of visual per-formance. For them, the world is an alien, confusing, and frightening place that can't be effectively addressed in any "normal" way.

Many hyperactive children, for instance, see the world as two-dimen-sional rather than three-dimensional. Objects in their environment appear flat to them, and they don't visually "feel" them. When you look at a house plant or a vase, you can easily grasp its form and location, but a hyperactive child can't, and thus he or she has an overwhelming urge to grasp the object physically—often with disastrous results. What looks like a behavior problem—"Johnny's out of control, he's like a bull in a china shop"—is actually the child's way of accommodating to a world in which space and form are distorted. Johnny can't locate objects with his visual system, so he uses his motor system. He's not bad, or wild; in fact, he's being perfectly logical.

Hypoactive children, on the other hand, react to their visual problems by saying, in effect, "I give up." Like a person simultaneously being told to turn left, turn right, go straight, and go backward, these children attempt to deal with a barrage of conflicting messages by doing nothing at all. These are the wallflowers, the kids who sit in the back of the class and hope they won't be noticed, and the children who sit on the sidelines as spectators. They're not lazy, or obstinate; rather, they've learned that they're likely to fail or even get into trouble by trying to act on the distorted visual data they receive.

To autistic children, the world can appear even more alien and unwelcoming, because their visual systems are far more impaired. Well-known autistic author Donna Williams, for example, remembers how walls would ripple and shimmer when she looked at them. Other autistic people experience "white-outs" and "black-outs," or say that looking at people directly is like looking "through a bowl of jelly."

These problems stem from deficits in the ambient vision processes involved in peripheral vision. Autistic and other disabled children often have perfectly normal focal vision—the central vision that allows us to identify objects when we look straight at them. In other words, they have no problem with the "What is it?" function. The problem lies instead with ambient vision, which involves the entire field of vision and tells us about the location of objects in space—the "Where is it?" function (more about this in Chapter 2).

When ambient vision is functioning properly, the eyes work as a team, producing separate but overlapping images. This allows us to see in three dimensions, and to accurately judge distance and movement. In patients with autism or related disabilities, we typically see two types of altered vision:

- "Tunnel vision" or compressed vision (hyperconvergence), in which the field of vision is constricted to a relatively small circle. Focusing only on what they see in this "tunnel," people with compressed vision view the world in two dimensions and cannot accurately judge distance or motion. In some cases, the world appears to be collapsing in on them.[1]

- "Alternating" vision (hypoconvergence or visual disparity), in which the eyes see two different images with no overlap. The person who exhibits hypoconvergence is basically seeing two dissimilar and competing views of the world. The result can be compared with viewing a movie with frames that are passing too slowly to give the illusion of continuous movement, and thus experiencing the sensation of a flickering rather than a steady picture. In some cases, we see the opposite effect, with images seeming to move too fast and producing a continuous blur.

Either compressed or alternating vision causes severe stress, not just to the visual system but to the body as a whole. Children with impaired ambient vision have trouble balancing, moving in a coordinated way, standing and walking correctly, and even knowing where their bodies end and the outside world begins. Often they cannot integrate space and time, and thus any motion in their environment—a tossed ball, a frolicking dog, a person approaching them—can seem unpredictable or even frightening. Lost in a world that makes no sense, unable to determine the boundaries of "me" and "other," they develop seemingly bizarre behaviors to compensate. These behaviors are evidence of a receptive, not an expressive, problem, and they are logical responses on the part of children with autism or related disabilities to sensory input that is incomprehensible.

Many autistic individuals walk on their toes, toe in when they walk, "stim" with their hands, or touch walls as they move through a room. All of these behaviors stem from their inability to handle both themselves and space simultaneously. To orient themselves, they flap their hands or touch objects, providing sensory input that tells them where they are in space. Their toe-walking tells us that they are insecure, and want to "hold on" to the ground as long as possible.

Autistic children also tend to rely on the more primitive senses of smell, touch, and taste. It's not unusual, for instance, to see an autistic child or adult sniff a toy, much like an infant would. This is because the information

Avoiding motion sickness

As a child, did you ever spin around and around until you felt nauseated, distressed, or even ready to vomit? That feeling is motion sickness, a natural reaction that occurs when we accelerate and lose control. One of the interesting things about autistic children is that many of them can spin endlessly without experiencing this reaction.

To understand why, it's useful to think about figure skaters and ballet dancers. Like us, these performers experience motion sickness. In order to do spins, they must consciously overcome this sensation. To accomplish this, they learn to "spot"—that is, to reduce their eye movements by fixing on a point in the audience and moving their heads, not their eyes. By giving priority to their focal vision system, and suppressing other visual and vestibular input, they avoid the symptoms of motion sickness.

For skaters and ballet dancers, this is a conscious act. Autistic individuals, on the other hand, learn to suppress their ambient visual processes instinctively, because it's the only way they can survive under a constant barrage of confusing, conflicting, and distressing input.

this individual receives from the sense of smell is more reliable than what he or she is seeing.

Children with autism tend to look at other people from the corners of their eyes, not because they are aloof, but because monocular vision makes more sense than trying to interpret data from two eyes that aren't working together. In addition, they may find it impossible to look at other people while conversing, because they can't process visual and auditory information at the same time. (A similar phenomenon occurs when you are so involved in trying to process visual information—for instance, while driving in dangerous traffic—that you are effectively deaf to another person's conversation. For many autistic children, life is always like this, and processing information from one sensory channel can be so difficult that it becomes necessary for them to block out all other competing stimuli.) In addition, autistic children may rock forward and backward, or wiggle their fingers in front of their faces, in order to experience depth perception.

In many respects an autistic child's world is like a carnival funhouse—a constant cascade of images that make no sense. If you are ever in one of these houses, study your own reactions and note how similar they are to that of an autistic child. Your instincts will be much the same: to walk cautiously, to touch surfaces because you can't tell where they are by looking, to turn or tilt your head in an attempt to make more sense of what you're seeing. For you, however, the experience will be temporary. For autistic children, it is permanent, unless they can find a path out through therapy.

The loss of "body sense"—that is, the knowledge of where the body ends and the outside world begins— isn't confined just to the people we label as autistic.

At one time, I worked in a residential home for individuals with emotional dysfunction, where one teenaged resident, Lacy, routinely asked staff members to pinch her. At first, I ignored her request. Eventually, however, puzzled by the urgency of her request, I reached out and pinched her.

"Thank you," Lacy said. When I asked her why she wanted me to pinch her, she replied, "because I can't feel where my body is."

While a psychiatrist might have interpreted Lacy's desire for pinching as an emotional symptom, in reality it was purely a physiological one. When I pinched her, I created a form of sensory input she could interpret, allowing her to feel secure and to know her physical place in her universe.

Similarly, autistic children who pinch or slap themselves often do so because they desperately need a form of sensory data that their brains can process, in order to "find" themselves in space. We can use behavior modification to reduce these behaviors, but it makes far more sense to understand them, and to correct the underlying visual dysfunction that creates the behaviors in the first place.

It's crucial to identify and correct the visual problems of children as quickly as possible, because these problems have a snowballing effect. The child who can't locate "self," other people, or objects in space increasingly focuses inwardly, missing out on crucial interactions with the environment. As a result, the child falls still further behind, with each missed milestone making it more difficult to catch up.

When we correct the initial visual problems that hold back development, we can then go back and revisit missed developmental stages. The result, often, is a remarkable reduction in symptoms, and a concurrent blossoming of intellectual, social, and communicative skills. Two cases will help to illustrate this point, both of them involving children whose visual dysfunction resulted in early disruption of the grasp-and-release skills that normally develop as a result of interaction between an infant's eyes and hands.

The first case involved a seven-year-old girl named Mattie, who briefly looked at objects when I handed them to her, but would not grasp them—a skill she should have mastered at 15 to 17 weeks of age. Instead, she would simply let an object lie in her palm. In order to stimulate Mattie's visual learning, we began by patterning her hands to grip, and then used startle procedures to stimulate her visual attention. Eventually, she learned to grasp a ball, and then to catch it easily.

Frank, also seven, would not toss a beanbag when asked to throw it into a basket, instead continuing to clutch it in his hand. When I demonstrated the skill, he still did not toss the beanbag, but instead walked over to the basket, and placed the beanbag in it. In Frank's case, a severe lack of depth perception led to early stunting of his visual-motor development, making it difficult for him to release an object (a developmental skill that actually follows grasping). When we addressed his impaired depth perception with ambient prism lenses and vision therapy, he was able to move more easily in three-dimensional space, and could successfully learn this skill and related ones. This was a first step in getting Frank's development back on track, and it quickly led to improvements in communicative and social skills.

It is important to note that while children and even adults can catch up on missed developmental stages, this doesn't mean that patients are "cured." In some cases, the results are so dramatic that children once diagnosed as having emotional disorders or pervasive developmental disorder (PDD) or high-functioning autism no longer qualify for those diagnoses. (For instance, one nonverbal four-year-old came to me labeled as having PDD. Within three months of starting vision therapy, he had language and began to function well. Six months after he started, his

One of my favorite cases involves a little boy I'll call Jay. At the age of six, Jay hardly ever spoke. He looked at books from the corner of his eye, and turned his head to one side when he rode a tricycle.

When he came to my office, Jay was tense and tearful, and ran away several times as I asked him to play games, catch a ball, and work on puzzles. But I gained a number of clues as I evaluated him. For instance, he initially refused to stack donut rings on a pyramid, throwing the pieces around the room. When I put a pair of ambient prism lenses on him, however, he immediately picked up the rings and placed them correctly on the pyramid. He exhibited the same pattern when I asked him to place wooden shapes in a puzzle board.

I prescribed prism lenses for Jay, and when they arrived two weeks later, his mother tried them on him. Before that day, he'd done simple puzzles slowly and with effort, matching the pieces to the pictures on the puzzle backing. "On that day, with glasses," his mother told me, "he sat down and put together five puzzles in quick succession. He placed the pieces around the edges, matching to colors and pictures for the first time. The next day he began putting two pieces together in his hands and completed the puzzles on the floor without any backing as a guide."

That was just the start of Jay's transformation. Soon, he began looking at books normally, instead of glancing at them from the corners of his eyes. He also started to look straight ahead when he ran or rode a tricycle.

Jay eventually graduated to another pair of prism lenses, and began a program of therapy to improve his self-awareness and aid him in using both sides of his body in a coordinated way. His progress was remarkable: he began touching people's faces, hugging others spontaneously, making eye contact, and showing an interest in other people's activities. His mother reported, only five months after Jay put on his first pair of glasses, "He now jabbers almost constantly and frequently uses full, meaningful sentences." He became toilet trained after many years of unsuccessful effort, and learned to spell, write words and numbers, read sentences and books out loud, and answer social questions.

Jay still has many developmental problems, and needs a variety of therapies. It's likely that he will be disabled, to some degree, for the rest of his life. But the huge strides he made during vision therapy are giving him a far better chance of leading a joyful and productive life.

parents took him to his neurologist, who said that he no longer qualified for a diagnosis of PDD.) In most cases, however, the patients remain disabled, because visual dysfunction is only one facet of their problem. But because vision is so key to performance, these individuals—despite the fact that they are still disabled—are able to open up to a new world of friends, family, and social and academic achievement that was once closed to them.

The improvement each patient experiences will depend, of course, on the patient's innate resilience and ability to change. It will also depend quite a bit on the person's motivation. Interestingly, patients with autism or other severe disabilities are often far more motivated, once they recognize the effects of prism lenses, than are very high-functioning patients with only minor impairments. The latter, because of their high adaptability, often learn to work successfully within the framework of their visual impairment, as illustrated by the case of a CEO who came to me for a visual perceptual consultation. When I asked him to read, he performed slowly and laboriously. I placed yoked prisms over his reading glasses, and he instantly began reading easily at a faster pace. His reaction was quite a surprise. He took off the glasses and said, "I don't want them… You're making my eyes move faster than I can think."

Most severely disabled patients, in contrast, find daily life a constant struggle, and they will instinctively grasp for the solutions we can offer them. Even patients who are withdrawn and nonverbal often react powerfully to prism lenses, work willingly at therapy, and make great progress.

Research shows the benefits of vision therapy

Successful case studies are compelling, and exciting for both doctors and parents, but the medical community likes to see proof of a therapy's effectiveness. So, to test the benefits of vision therapy, our institute has conducted several scientific studies over the past decade.

For the first study,[2] we recruited 14 autistic children between the ages of 4 and 15, and observed their head positions and body posture as they watched TV, walked on a balance beam, or caught a ball. We evaluated their posture, facial expressions, and head positions during these activities. Next, we analyzed the children's reactions when we gave them either correct ambient prism lenses or "wrong" lenses (which either interfered with visual performance or did not alter it at all).

We found that children wearing either no lenses or "wrong" lenses continued to perform poorly, while those wearing corrective lenses showed immediate and often dramatic changes, such as the following:

- Children who previously tilted their heads were much more likely to hold their heads erect, in the correct position, while wearing the lenses.

- In the ball-catching task, the children actively caught the ball far more often, and scored far fewer misses or "passive catches."

- The children's facial expressions changed markedly when they wore the glasses, becoming much less tense.

It's important to note that we saw these remarkable changes *after only a few minutes*. Ambient prism lenses are only the first step in vision therapy, and the changes that occur with the glasses are often minuscule compared with the exponential long-term improvement we see as we enable children to catch up on missed milestones.

In a second study,[3] which we conducted in 1998, we followed a group of 18 autistic children for a longer period after they received their ambient prism lenses. Although the children received no therapy, they exhibited a significant decrease in behavior problems over the first two months in response to the glasses alone. These benefits began to fade slightly at four months—just as we'd predicted, because prism lenses and vision therapy must work hand-in-hand to create permanent changes.

The successes brought about by vision therapy are immensely gratifying for those of us who are privileged to see them first-hand. I've seen children who were locked in their own secret world begin to enjoy people and experiences. I've seen nonverbal children suddenly begin to speak, and learning-disabled children learn to read and write and spell. And I've seen gains, large and small, made by children whose doctors said their symptoms were "untreatable."

All of these changes were possible because I listened to my patients, and to the messages they sent me with their "stims," their toe-walking, their hyperactivity, and their other adaptations to their visual problems. This is why I tell parents and professionals to remember that *the behavior is not the problem—it is the key to the solution.* That solution is right in front of us, if we take the time to listen, look, and learn, and if we fully believe in the ability of our patients to change and grow.

Jacqueline Goldwyn Kingon, the mother of a young man with Asperger Syndrome who is now an accomplished musician, recently wrote eloquently in the *New York Times* about her son's early years:

> It did not matter to me that he had just been thrown out of a nursery school for retarded children because of too many tantrums. It did not matter that competing doctors identified him as either brain-injured, autistic, learning disabled, developmentally delayed or emotionally disturbed while denigrating and disputing the diagnoses from rival associates in other therapeutic disciplines. I saw ability where they saw disability.[4]

When we do the same, and nurture the glimmers of ability we see in our patients, we can truly empower them to "see through new eyes."

Notes

1 Ivar Lovaas was one of the first researchers to report on tunnel vision in autistic children. He used the term "stimulus overselectivity" to describe attention to only one aspect of the environment.

2 Kaplan, M., Carmody, D. and Gaydos, A. (1998) "Postural orientation modifications in autism in response to ambient lenses." *Child Psychiatry and Human Development 27*, 2, 81–91.

3 Kaplan, M., Edelson, S.M. and Seip, J.L. (1998) "Behavioural changes in autistic individuals as a result of wearing ambient transitional prism lenses." *Child Psychiatry and Human Development 29*, 65–76.

4 Kingon, Jacqueline Goldwyn (2004) "Beautiful music." *New York Times*, 7 November.

CHAPTER 2

Prism Lenses and Vision Therapy: Overview and Historical Perspective

Optometrist Leo Manas once said in a lecture, "There is no professional who has more power to change a person's life than his optometrist doing his job properly." Professionals who specialize in behavioral optometry know the truth of this statement. I've seen hundreds of my patients instantly transformed by the effects of prism lenses, and I've seen these transformations translate into lasting and life-changing improvements when these patients undergo vision therapy.

Why is vision therapy so effective in changing behavior and improving performance? To answer that question, it is first necessary to discuss the shortcomings of the traditional medical model of vision. This medical model considers visual dysfunction as a *structural* problem, involving the recognition of forms. A child can't see the blackboard, so he is given glasses for nearsightedness. A middle-aged person can't see small print, so she receives a prescription for magnifying lenses. An elderly person's vision is blurred by a cataract, so his anatomical lens is replaced by a man-made one. This is a static concept: an eye has a defect, so something optical is done to correct it.

A newer and much more accurate paradigm—the developmental model—recognizes that vision is a *dynamic* process, which controls the action of the entire body and, in turn, is influenced by feedback from other sensory systems. Vision is not a static receptor of information, according to this model, but an interactive one.

A key difference between the medical and developmental models of vision is that while there are two visual systems, vision professionals trained under the medical model primarily address the structural problems that occur in only one of these: the *focal* vision system. This is the high-resolution central vision that allows us to identify objects, and it is the system that can be impaired by cataracts, refraction errors, and other "hardware" problems. Focal vision, limited to only a few degrees of the visual field, operates largely under conscious control and makes it possible for us to see colors and identify stable features of our surroundings. Defects of the focal vision system typically are treated either surgically or with corrective lenses that compensate for the eye's inability to focus correctly.

Developmental optometrists recognize the importance of focal vision problems, but they also recognize that severe problems can arise in the second system that allows us to interpret our visual world: the *ambient* visual system. Ambient vision, also referred to as peripheral vision, encompasses the entire visual field. It is a lower-resolution system that operates largely on a non-conscious level, and allows us to rapidly identify where we are and what is happening in our environment. While focal vision is largely static, ambient vision is dynamic, integrating with other sensory systems to update us constantly about our changing world—and it works correctly only if the "software" of the neural system is intact. Table 2.1 shows the differences between the two vision systems.

Identifying deficits in ambient vision is crucial, because this system is key to defining both our self-image and our view of our world. Right now, for example, your ambient vision is sending you a constant stream of data about the location of your body in space, and the location of other people or objects—in addition to telling you how quickly they are moving, and in what direction. If someone walks up to you, your focal vision will tell you who the person is—but your ambient vision will quickly transmit critical cues about the person's changing "body language," how close he or she is to you, and whether you should be relaxed or alarmed by the encounter. If you move to another spot, your ambient vision will tell you where you're going, and update your position in relation to doors, chairs, tables, and walls. Turn on the television, and your ambient vision will allow you to watch the moving picture, coordinate that picture with the sound from the TV, and form both into a coherent whole. It will also allow you to watch the TV while still being aware of a friend passing by outside the window, or a cat creeping up beside you.

Table 2.1 Ambient vs. focal vision

Ambient vision	Focal vision
"Where am I/Where is it?" function	"What is it?" (object recognition) function
Dynamic (kinetic)—identifies movement, change	Static—identifies stable features of surroundings
Low-resolution non-color vision (rods)	High-resolution color vision (cones)
Involves entire visual field	Involves only central vision—limited to central two degrees of visual field (fovea)
Not degraded at night	Degraded at night
Largely non-conscious	Largely conscious
Integrates with other sensory systems	Works in isolation
Is largely learned, and thus can be greatly enhanced through a program of visual management	Is innate rather than learned

Disrupt this ambient visual system, and simple activities that you take for granted—from climbing stairs, to watching TV, to talking with another person—can become highly difficult and stressful ordeals. Objects will appear closer or farther away than they really are, causing you to be clumsy or disoriented. Other people's body language may be hard to read, making social situations frightening. Catching a football, navigating a crowded hallway, or driving a car can be terrifying. If the disruption is severe, even identifying where your own body ends, and the outside world begins, can become impossible.

Because ambient visual problems affect the "software" of the visual system, we can't address them effectively with surgery or standard glasses. However, a crucial aspect of ambient vision is that, unlike focal vision, it is largely *learned* and thus can respond to intervention in the form of vision therapy. This fact, overlooked by much of the medical profession, has enormous implications for professionals in the field of vision.

The earliest clues that the visual circuitry adapts to environmental changes came in the early 1960s, when Harvard researchers David Hubel and Torsten Wiesel altered the eyesight of very young cats by blurring their vision with contact lenses, patching one eye, or causing strabismus. When Hubel and Wiesel autopsied the cats later, they discovered that the neurons associated with binocular vision had atrophied. Similarly, Austin Riesen found that binocular cells in the brain cannot be stimulated by input from one eye alone; his research showed that "synchronous inputs from the two eyes are required during early development if normal binocular function is to appear."[1] These findings provided definitive proof that early visual disruption changes the brain's response to visual stimuli, and thus that experience alters what a cat (or a human) actually sees.

Equally important, studies show that if given intensive training, animals subjected to early visual disruption can learn ambient visual skills—a finding that is equally true for humans. Moreover, we now know that the concept of a "critical period," after which visual problems are not correctable, is inaccurate. Vision therapy works best with young children, but studies show that remarkable improvement can occur in adults as well.[2] This is consistent with animal studies by von Noorden, Van Sluyters, and Pettigrew, all of whom found that visual anomalies due to early deprivation could be completely reversed, well after any supposed "critical period" had elapsed.[3]

This is no surprise, when you consider that ambient visual processes have evolved specifically to allow us to deal with an ever-changing environment. The visual skills needed to succeed in the jungle are different from those needed to cope in downtown New York City, or on a sailboat in choppy seas. Similarly, the visual skills needed to survive as an elementary-school student are different from those needed to survive as a baby or toddler. An organism that can adapt visually to changing environments is an organism that is likely to survive.

Indeed, constant adaptive changes occur in the human visual system, particularly during youth and early adulthood. The baby who reaches for a rattle and shakes it, the toddler who learns to successfully stack six blocks, or the preschooler who practices cutting out shapes with scissors is experiencing a continuous feedback loop that refines both motor skills and ambient vision. Similarly, the teenager learning to drive a car in traffic, or the athlete practicing a tennis backhand, is honing ambient visual skills.

While there are optimal periods for training visual skills, we now know that visual learning continues throughout life. Studies reveal that adults who regain their vision after a long period of blindness are able to identify objects (a focal skill), but are unable to deal with the spatial organization of objects (an ambient skill). With practice, however, these adults are able to regain, refine, and improve their ambient skills. The same is true for patients of any age who have poor ambient vision as a result of neurological deficits. The visual skills of these individuals are not irrevocably lost but merely dormant, often because they have shut down visual systems in order to cope with a confusing world. When we allow these patients to make sense of their environment, by altering their perception with prism lenses and consolidating their gains with vision therapy, we create permanent neurological changes that translate into a new view of the world.

Who needs vision therapy?

Even among the "normal" population, vision deficits are a surprisingly common problem. For example, a report of the American Optometric Association notes, "The New York State Vision Screening Battery probes oculomotor, binocular, accommodative, and visual perceptual function. Testing of 1634 children with this battery revealed a failure rate of 53 percent." Between 4 and 8 percent of school-age children exhibit strabismus, while as many as 8 percent are affected by amblyopia, and studies of adults show that convergence insufficiency occurs in 15 percent of them.[4] In short, large numbers of individuals with no apparent ocular problems exhibit "hidden" performance-altering visual deficits, most often involving ambient visual processes.

In special populations—including individuals with autism, other developmental delays, or learning disabilities—the rate of vision problems is astronomically higher. Here are some of the findings of researchers:

- Scharre and Creedon evaluated 34 autistic children between the ages of 2 and 11. None of the children had overt ocular disease, dysmorphic features, or seizure disorders that could affect visual function. The researchers found that 21 percent of the children were strabismic at far distances, and 18 percent at near distances. In addition, only 14.7 percent of the children exhibited voluntary pursuit movements. Thirty-one exhibited atypical optokinetic nystagmus response (the alternating smooth pursuit and saccades normally elicited when an individual looks at passing objects while spinning, riding in a car, etc.), including delayed onset, short duration, gaze avoidance, or stereotypic behavior.[5]

- Denis and colleagues evaluated ten children with autism and found that six of them exhibited strabismus. (The researchers also found a surprising rate of focal vision problems, including hypermetropia and astigmatism.) They conclude that the problems they detected "can lead to amblyopia (chronic visual disorders) with the risk of functional loss of vision."[6]

- A 1990 study in which I participated found that 50 percent of a group of 34 autistic children undergoing optometric evaluation exhibited strabismus. In addition, using a large database containing information on more than 7000 children with "classical" autism, we found that 20 percent of their parents mentioned "crossed eyes" as a symptom.[7]

- A review of Special Olympics physicals determined that 25 percent of developmentally disabled individuals exhibited strabismus.[8]

- A recent screening of 1539 adults with intellectual disabilities found that 44.1 percent exhibited strabismus.[9]

- Granet and colleagues reviewed the charts of 266 patients, and found that nearly 16 percent of patients with attention deficit hyperactivity disorder had convergence insufficiency problems—more than three times as many as would normally be expected.[10]

- Grisham reported that children with reading disabilities showed a greater than 50 percent prevalence of visual deficiencies in accommodation, fusional vergence or gross convergence, compared with non-learning-disabled peers.[11]

- A recent study of visual attention skills found that children with autism have marked difficulty in disengaging their attention from one visual stimulus in order to focus on another. "Indeed," Landry and Bryson reported, "in 20 percent of trials they remained fixated on the first of two competing stimuli for the entire eight-second trial duration." This behavior, the researchers note, is similar to that of normal two-month-olds, who are unable to switch attention readily from one visual stimulus to another.[12]

Clearly, visual deficits are a serious and largely undetected problem among special populations. These deficits severely impair the ability of affected individuals to define their own bodies and the world around them, and to integrate visual input with input from other sensory systems—all skills crucial to functioning physically, academically, and emotionally in a visual world.

The effectiveness of prism lenses and vision therapy

Despite the high incidence of vision abnormalities in the population, professionals interested in offering a visual management program incorporating the use of prism lenses may find that they encounter skepticism from colleagues. There are two reasons for this: a general ignorance about vision therapy itself, and, more specifically, a lack of awareness about the use and purpose of prism lenses.

Vision therapy is still considered by many professionals to be "experimental," even though it has been successfully employed for a century and has a proven track record of success. A full discussion of the literature supporting vision therapy is beyond the scope of this book, but for those unfamiliar with this literature, a 2003 position paper by the American Optometric Association (AOA) summarizes more than 150 studies documenting the beneficial effects of vision therapy in correcting abnormal eye movements, ameliorating accommodative dysfunctions, and remediating binocular vision disorders.[13] Research findings cited by the AOA include:

Effects of therapy on eye movement

In a study by Wold, Pierce, and Keddington of 100 consecutive optometric vision therapy patients, only 6 percent of children passed a test of eye movement performance prior to therapy. Following therapy, 96 percent of the children were able to pass.[14]

Effects of therapy on accommodation deficits

In a similar study, Wold *et al.* reported on 100 children who underwent accommodative vision therapy. The children showed an 80 percent rate of improvement in accommodative amplitude and 76 percent in accommodative facility.[15]

Effects of therapy on convergence insufficiency

Cooper and Duckman reviewed an extensive body of research on the use of vision therapy for convergence insufficiency, and reported that 95 percent of the patients in the studies they reviewed responded favorably to vision therapy. The AOA report also notes, "Dalzie reported on 100 convergence insufficiency patients who did not meet Sheard's criterion [a test of fusional convergence ability], and were given a program of vision therapy. After vision therapy, clinical findings were again assessed and 84 percent of the patients successfully met Sheard's criterion. Eighty-three percent of the patients reported they had symptoms of discomfort or loss of efficiency prior to treatment. Only 7 percent reported these symptoms after therapy."[16]

Effects of therapy on strabismus

A research review by Flom revealed an overall functional cure rate of 50 percent for strabismics receiving vision therapy, with exotropia responding better than esotropia.[17] Ludlam evaluated 149 unselected strabismics who received vision therapy and reported a 73 percent overall success rate using strict outcome criteria.[18]

These and numerous other studies show conclusively that vision therapy greatly aids patients with visual disorders, and is particularly helpful for those with disorders severe enough to interfere with academic, social, and communicative skills. It is my experience that professionals whose visual management programs incorporate the use of ambient prism lenses, one of the most powerful tools we have to improve vision, can greatly enhance these benefits.

Overview: yoked prism lenses as a treatment modality

The use of prisms in glasses is, of course, nothing new. Conventional eye care professionals often use prisms in one lens, in order to compensate for ocular muscle imbalances. This is consistent with the medical model of visual defects as an issue of mechanics—that is, a hardware problem. The purpose of ambient prism lenses, however, is not to compensate for a mechanical defect, but rather to actually *alter perception* in ways that cause patients to reorganize their visual processes. In short, ambient prism lenses are a neural intervention, which addresses the "software" of the visual system.

All lenses are effectively optical prisms. The farther from the optical center a light ray stimulates a lens, the more the ray displaces the perceived image. However, the effect of a prism is not limited to displacement. The prismatic visual field appears compressed at the base (flat edge) and expanded on the apex (thin edge), because light rays are deflected differently according to the direction of the rays and the magnitude of the prism.

Ambient (yoked) prism lenses consist of prisms of equal diopter before each eye. Both prisms are oriented in the same direction: either base-up, base-down, base-left, or base-right. The effect of wearing yoked prisms is to deflect peripheral light rays, shifting space in a manner that dramatically alters the patient's view of the external world. Base-down yoked prisms displace the visual system upward, and near objects are amplified while distant ones are reduced. Base-up prisms displace the visual system downward, and near objects are reduced while distant ones are amplified. Base-left prisms make objects appear farther away on the left, and nearer on the right, while base-right prisms have the opposite effect. Ambient prism lenses cause a transformation in different planes, forcing patients to actively reorganize visual processes in order to achieve homeostasis.

The behavioral changes caused by this alteration of perception often are instantaneous and dramatic. Patients with autism or related disabilities have spent a lifetime developing strategies to compensate for their visual deficits. By the time they arrive at the optometrist's office, these strategies—eye turns, postural warps, self-stimulating behaviors, etc.—are habitual and ingrained. Ambient prism lenses instantly create a new visual world, in which those adaptive mechanisms are no longer either necessary or relevant. As a result, patients must rapidly re-awaken previously suppressed visual processes, in order to make sense of their altered surroundings. In effect, the perceptual changes brought about by yoked

From skepticism to tradition

As I mention in this chapter, the use of ambient prism lenses is considered new and even radical by many traditional eye care professionals. What is interesting in this regard is that the standard use of *any* type of lenses, including the lenses now prescribed every day for nearsighted or farsighted patients, was considered unscientific or even dangerous by ophthalmologists until relatively recently. This was true even though "the common folk" began using such lenses as early as the 13th century.

The refusal of ophthalmologists to accept the use of lenses led them to adopt many odd theories about the causes and treatment of vision problems. For instance, in the 1840s, an ophthalmologist named Mackenzie noted that students frequently suffered from a form of eyestrain, which he dubbed asthenopia. If you were an 18-year-old male student at Oxford at this time, and displayed symptoms including slight light sensitivity, a tendency to frown, good distance sight, and stress during near-point tasks, you would quite likely be sent to Dr. Mackenzie, whose diagnosis would be asthenopia. The cause? According to Mackenzie and other prominent ophthalmologists at the time, it was excessive masturbation, which they believed caused ocular weakness. The treatment? In addition to being told to give up reading, patients were sometimes subjected to cauterization of the urethra!

Patients who wanted to avoid such a fate avoided ophthalmologists, and instead obtained convex lenses from opticians. When they did, their symptoms were reduced and in some cases eliminated. It wasn't until 40 years later, however, at the Wills Eye Clinic in Philadelphia, that the first pair of convex lenses for asthenopia was prescribed in an ophthalmologic setting.

My point in offering this history lesson is not to disparage traditional ophthalmologists, but rather to point out that in the field of vision care, it typically takes decades for new and beneficial developments to become accepted practice. The same is true, moreover, in every field of medicine. Getting the medical community to accept new ideas takes more than proof—it also takes time.

prisms—which include a perception of increased curvature, displacement of objects, and a tilting of the meridian planes—require patients to "recalibrate" their visual systems, using skills that previously were suppressed.

For a fascinating look at how the distortions caused by prism lenses cause the viewer to reorganize and reintegrate visual processes, I recommend *Living in a World Transformed*, a classic work by Hubert Dolezal.[19] Dolezal, a psychology professor, experimented with prism lenses that reversed the image seen by his eyes, initially making the world appear upside down. Within days, however, he was able to function competently, and to perceive the world as right-side-up, in spite of the reversed image his retinas received. Dolezal's experiments, and similar experiments conducted by George Stratton before him, revealed that the brain can reorganize visual processes in adaptation to new input—whether this input is normalized by facilitative prism lenses, or distorted by disruptive lenses. (Both types of lenses are used in vision therapy, as I will discuss in Chapter 4.)

A brief history of prism lenses

While the use of yoked prism lenses is fairly new, the historical groundwork for the use of these lenses was laid more than a century ago. In 1859, Albrecht Von Grafe theorized that asthenopia stems not only from abnormalities of the muscles that accommodate the eye for form recognition, but also from abnormalities of the extrinsic muscles that direct our attention to what we are looking for. (These six pairs of muscles, which turn the eyes to find objects, are controlled by the third, fourth and sixth cranial nerves.) In short, he was the first to equate dynamic *aiming* deficits as well as static *focusing* deficits as a cause for asthenopia.

In the 1920s, A.M. Skeffington, considered the "father of behavioral optometry," built on this foundation when he pioneered the concept that vision was learned, and could be improved through intervention. Skeffington demonstrated that deficits in *centering*—that is, the ability to know where another object is in relationship to the viewer—were a cause of asthenopia, a radical idea at the time. He also advanced the concept of vision as a process that emerges from the interaction of spatial, motor, and intellectual function, and involves four sub-processes (see Figure 2.1): centering (the "Where is it?" function), identification (the "What is it?" function), antigravity (relating to balance and posture in space), and

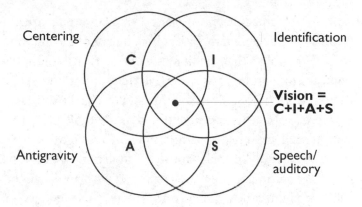

Figure 2.1: Skeffington's four circles

speech/auditory processes (the ability to label what we see). Skeffington was one of the first practitioners to use lenses as a learning tool, saying that "lenses are the fastest way to change a person."

In the late 1940s, optometrists began routinely using developmental glasses for prevention of asthenopia as well as certain conditions of myopia. Developmental glasses use convex lenses of low magnitude, making print appear farther away and requiring less innervation for the eyes to converge, thus keeping the focusing system relaxed. Optometrists prescribing these glasses found that they could prevent asthenopia and, in many cases, myopia.

Although the use of lenses has thus been part of developmental optometry for many years, the use of ambient prism lenses is a relatively recent development. It was in the 1970s at the Gesell Institute that I was introduced to yoked prisms, a concept pioneered by Dr. Bruce Wolff, who was successfully using large-magnitude yoked prisms to address behavioral and learning problems in children and adults. At the Gesell Institute, Richard Apell and John Streff shared with us how large-magnitude yoked prisms create a distorted illusion of the outer world, forcing patients to become aware of their environment in a new way that leads them to reorganize their manner of thinking, moving, and feeling. Apell and his colleagues emphasized, however, that vision therapy was a necessary adjunct to the use of prism lenses, if patients were to secure meaning and understanding from the changes the lenses created.

I began using low-magnitude therapeutic lenses in my own practice around 1972, at a time when very few practitioners were doing so. While Apell and Streff had emphasized the use of yoked prisms to disrupt visual processes, I hit upon the concept of using low-magnitude yoked prisms not as a disruptive device but rather as a direct means of facilitating vision. My initial work revealed that facilitative yoked prisms could markedly reduce symptoms of learning disabilities, anxiety, and motion sickness.

The seminal work of John Szentágothai and Michael Arbib, authors of *Conceptual Models of Neural Organization* (the outgrowth of an MIT research program) influenced me greatly at this time.[20] Szentágothai and Arbib wrote that we must analyze the brain from an action-oriented point of view, saying, "We must not only understand how neural networks can enable an animal to interact with its world, but also must understand how those networks can be structured so as to allow efficient updating with experience." Szentágothai and Arbib emphasized that the brain is not static. It seeks homeostasis—a return to what it considers as normal—and to achieve that homeostasis, it constantly interacts with its environment and updates its information. Through its hierarchical feedback and "feed-forward" loops, and its correlation of input from different senses, it seeks to explore, adapt to, and thus control its environment. With the use of the right lenses, I realized, I could influence this adaptive process and, in turn, the behavior of an individual.

The effects of yoked prism lenses on motion sickness were of particular interest to me at this point in my career, as they revealed how these lenses could affect the feedback cycles that influence visual and vestibular processing. Early on I realized, and the literature reaffirmed to me, that the nervous system works much like a telephone system, in that incoming and outgoing "calls" are made from one sensing system to the other. This means that while vestibular input can alter visual processing (as is the case of motion sickness, in which a disturbance of the vestibular system in the inner ear causes disturbances in visual perception), the reverse is also true: changes in the visual system can influence the vestibular system. In testing this concept, I indeed found that the use of directive yoked prisms could stabilize eye movements, which in turn could stabilize the vestibular system. This finding, moreover, was true for patients of all ages.

One amusing example of this involved a young learning-disabled man named Carl, who initially suffered from motion sickness to such a degree that he would vomit even during short car rides. I provided Carl with yoked prisms, which relieved his headaches and stomach aches, and completely eliminated his motion sickness. Shortly afterward, during a long car trip, he was quite comfortable, but his mother developed severe motion sickness. Borrowing Carl's glasses, she found that they cured her symptoms—but Carl, deprived of the glasses, once again became nauseated. As a result, the two spent the entire trip battling fiercely over who would get to wear the glasses!

As I continued working with yoked prism lenses, I found that many patients with severe anxiety—a problem generally believed at that time to be strictly psychogenic—had similar problems in integrating visual and vestibular input. These patients often responded wonderfully to yoked prisms, and my colleagues in the psychiatric community started sending me many patients suffering from anxiety. Often these patients displayed convergence insufficiency or convergence excess, along with poor resilience and saccadic eye movements.

The histories of patients suffering from severe anxiety typically involved childhood symptoms of motion sickness, evolving slowly into full-blown panic or anxiety disorder around the age of 30, at which time the patients typically consulted psychiatrists or psychologists. This pattern, which I saw over and over again in patients, opened my eyes to the concept that disorders labeled as "emotional" or "psychiatric" frequently stemmed in reality from correctable vision deficits.

One of the most dramatic experiences of my career, and one that permanently altered the course of my work, occurred at about this time. It involved a young woman whose full story is told in the book *Rickie*,[21] written by her father, psychiatrist Frederic Flach. At the age of 13, Rickie—a beautiful and highly intelligent child, but already considered "troubled"—developed symptoms labeled as schizophrenia. Transferred from one mental institution to another for a decade, Rickie failed to respond to drugs, electroshock, or psychotherapy. Each brief recovery ended abruptly in a catastrophic emotional meltdown, a bout of violent self-injury, or a suicide attempt. Rickie's father, a prominent psychiatrist, learned about my work from a mutual friend. He was skeptical—what could vision have to do with symptoms of schizophrenia?—but he was desperate, and willing to try anything. He asked me, "Can you help Rickie?" When I responded, "Visually or psychologically?" he replied, "Any way you can."

Rickie, while very cooperative, initially found my routine evaluation alarming. During my exam, she displayed gross nystagmoid movements. When I shined a light into her eyes, she reared back like a frightened animal. Instead of a normal retinal movement, she exhibited a scissor motion, and her visual acuity—which I'd tested earlier and found to be 20/30—instantly dropped to 20/200. In seconds, she'd shut down her visual system to the point where she was legally blind.

Intrigued by this response, I asked Rickie if an image persisted when she looked at it, or disappeared. She replied, "I can *make* it stay." Elaborating on her answer, she explained that if she looked at me for a minute, my image would start to disappear. However, she added, "If I get my willpower going, I can keep you in sight for a long time." I asked what happened to other people or objects in the room, and she said, "At first I see them, and you. Then, as I concentrate harder on seeing you, they get dimmer and dimmer, until I can't see them at all." Further testing revealed that Rickie had severely impaired depth perception, experienced difficulty maintaining stable vision in one eye, and had very little idea of where other objects, or even her own body, were in space.

Rickie, I discovered, had to use every ounce of her energy trying to compensate for severely impaired visual processes. When she was three, her father remembered, she'd suddenly become terrified one day while looking out a window, saying, "The trees are coming to the house. They're all coming in here." Most likely, this was the first sign of Rickie's catastrophic loss of depth perception, possibly triggered by earlier surgery to remove a forehead tumor. To compensate for the terrifying feeling that the world was closing in on her, she'd developed tunnel vision, protecting her from the terrors she saw but restricting her vision to disjointed snapshots with little context. (Imagine going through life viewing the world through two long tubes that block your peripheral vision, and you can begin to picture how disabling and frightening such a visual deficit is.)

Not surprisingly, Rickie experienced terrible difficulty in school, saying that words "crumbled" on the blackboard when she tried to read them. When stressed, she developed tunnel vision so extreme that her world appeared completely alien. In one incident, which resulted in her readmission to a psychiatric facility, she broke down in the classroom because "I could hardly see… The whole room looked dark… [the teacher's head] looked like it wasn't even connected to her body." Additional relapses occurred each time she tried to return to the classroom.

As part of my evaluation of Rickie, I asked her to walk on a balance beam. Each time, she fell off after about three steps. I then gave her a pair of base-down prism lenses to wear and a string of beads to hold in her hand, and asked her to walk on the beam again. She moved across the board effortlessly, with a broad smile on her face. The prisms expanded space for her, giving her more control over her environment, while the beads helped to "anchor" her and compensate for her lack of body awareness.

Rickie entered therapy, and her treatment took about one year. During that time she also underwent nutritional therapy and counseling at another facility, where an excellent staff made sure she followed the vision management plan I outlined. The results amazed all of us: relieved of her stressful and energy-sapping visual problems, and finally able to see the world as a whole rather than as a jumble of disconnected images, Rickie blossomed in front of our eyes. After ten years in institutions, she learned to cope on her own, went on to a career as a practical nurse, and married and had several children. "That Rickie was functionally blind is indisputable," her father commented in his book. "She had probably been visually disabled since the age of three, and it is conceivable that until that disability had been corrected, no form of treatment would have produced lasting results."

Dr. Flach and I later collaborated professionally in a research project that revealed that two-thirds of psychiatric patients suffer from some form of visual dysfunction, with the most serious deficits occurring in patients with schizophrenia, unipolar depression, or alcohol dependence. In our study, nearly 85 percent of patients with severe, chronic mental illness exhibited marked impairments in spatial organization due to visual impairments. Patients with the most severe vision problems exhibited the highest levels of social withdrawal, academic failure, and employment difficulties.[22]

Vision and behavioral symptoms: a chicken-or-egg question

Years ago, a group of researchers at New York University organized a study to track the eye movements of people with schizophrenia. Their goal was to see if abnormal saccades could be used as a marker for the disorder.

Rickie's father, Dr. Flach, invited me to watch their experiment. Observing the testing, I asked the head researcher a simple question: "If your research proves that saccadic eye movement dysfunction is a sign of schizophrenia, does that mean that if you can stop the saccadic eye movement dysfunction, your patient will no longer be schizophrenic?" My point was simple: they were looking at how *schizophrenia caused abnormal eye movements*, while I knew that *abnormal eye movements could cause many symptoms attributed to schizophrenia*—and that both the abnormal eye movements and the resulting symptoms could be altered by prism lenses and vision therapy.   .

My question threw the researcher for a loop. I explained that reha- bilitating eye movement dysfunctions was what I did for a living, and I invited him to my office for a first-hand demonstration of the effects of eye movements on behavior. When he arrived, my staff performed two tests—the Keystone Skills and Van Orden Star— which revealed that he had a global style and scanpath eye movements. In the ball play task he could not catch the ball, and he admitted that he was always the last one picked for a sports team in his youth.

I placed yoked base-up prisms on the researcher. When I threw the ball to him, he reached out and caught it easily. "What happened?" he asked. "I stabilized your eye movements," I told him. In his case, I said, minor visual impairments merely caused him difficulty in sports ("Where is the ball?"). The more severe impairments of people with mental illness, I explained, have much more debilitating effects ("Where am I?" "Why are the walls closing in on me?" "Why is the wallpaper pattern moving?"), and thus can cause symptoms up to and including schizophrenic behavior.

The researcher wondered how lenses would affect the eye-tracking movements his team was measuring, so I brought three pairs of yoked prism lenses to NYU (base-up, base-down, and placebo), color-coded so the researchers couldn't tell them apart. Dr. Flach offered to be a guinea pig for our test. We placed the base-down lenses on him first, and the researchers' print-out showed dysfunc- tional saccades. I then applied the placebo pair, and Dr. Flach's eye movements became smooth. When I gave him the base-up pair, his eye movement was highly stable.

The researcher's skeptical response was, "It's probably a learned response." So I said, "Let's retry the black pair" (which was the original base-down pair). When we did, the dysfunctional saccade instantly reappeared. I laughed and said jokingly, "I guess he doesn't retain well."

My demonstrations in my office and at NYU helped to convince the researchers that abnormal eye movements could indeed cause symptoms—and that with yoked prism lenses, we could alter both the eye movements and the symptoms themselves.

Vision therapy and the patient with autism

Rickie's remarkable response to prism lenses and therapy, and the results of my research with Dr. Flach, opened my eyes to the possibility that many other patients diagnosed as mentally ill could benefit from this approach. As a result, over time, I broadened my practice to include more and more patients with psychiatric disorders, including those with autism.

When I first began working with children on the autism spectrum, I detected the same pattern in them as I'd seen in Rickie. These children, overwhelmed by input their brains cannot interpret, often shut down their ambient vision to the point where many are functionally blind—even though, like Rickie, they have "normal" visual acuity. As a result, they stagnate developmentally. Non-disabled children experience constant cycles of growth and learning, with each cycle accompanied by a stage of disequilibrium (for instance, the "terrible twos") until new behaviors are integrated and a new stability is achieved. Autistic children, unable to move through these stages because of their sensory deficits, fall ever farther behind. They remain mired in a constant state of tension, unable to learn, refine, and consolidate new skills.

While impaired vision is not the only neurological problem these children exhibit, the dominant role of the visual system in learning and development makes impairment of this system particularly deleterious. As Arnold Gesell wrote, "The infant takes hold of the world with his eyes long before he does so with his hands—an extremely significant fact. During the first eight weeks of life the hands remain predominantly fisted, while the eyes and brain are busy with looking, staring, seeking, and, in a rudimentary manner, apprehending."[23] The child with autism cannot use his or her visual system efficiently to explore the world in this way, and must depend on the more rudimentary senses of touch, smell, or taste. This inefficient method makes the world immensely more difficult to understand, and leads to severe delays in development.

Many autistic children also display symptoms indicative of vestibular involvement. Although they cannot verbally describe how they feel, their vestibular dysfunction is quite apparent from their hypersensitivity to visual stimuli, fear of heights, and fear of movement. As I noted in the previous chapter, many autistic children respond to these problems by suppressing input from their vestibular and ambient visual systems and instead rely on focal vision, with the resulting effect that they do not experience motion sickness even in circumstances (such as spinning) in which they should. I have found over the years that when we address the visual deficits of these children, we see resulting improvements in vestibular function as well.

The vestibular system, moreover, is only one of multiple sensory modalities affected by ambient visual processes. In 40 years of working with autistic and other disabled patients, I have found that when we use prism lenses to retrain and reintegrate the visual system, we are not just restoring isolated visual skills. We are also, by extension, improving a patient's ability to reintegrate visual processes with other sensory systems—auditory, tactile, proprioceptive, gravitational—in order to achieve a new and higher level of performance. This is a key reason why therapy utilizing prism lenses can have such a profound effect not just on visual processes but also on behavior, communication, and social interaction.

Still another explanation for the benefits of vision therapy comes from research indicating that impaired visual ability causes the brain to use less efficient routes in processing stimuli—a problem that visual management can often overcome. In *The Emotional Brain*,[24] Joseph LeDoux notes how sensory stimuli initially travel a "low road" from the thalamus to the amygdala, which makes quick but rough judgments about how to respond. Simultaneously, the same information takes the "high road" from the thalamus to the cortex, which creates a much more accurate representation of the stimulus and sends this data to the amygdala, allowing the brain to make a more refined response. For instance, LeDoux notes, if you spot a long object that may be a snake or a stick, your immediate reaction (based on the "low road") will be to run. A split second later, the input routed through your visual cortex (the "high road") will allow you to refine your emotional response if the object proves to be harmless. Because people with autism shut down much of their higher visual processing, my hypothesis is that they bypass this "high road" and thus base much of their behavior upon inadequate input provided solely by the thalamic-amygdala pathway. This is a very inefficient system, leading to chronically inappropriate emotional and behavioral responses and leaving little energy for higher functions such as communication. When we reorganize brain processing through the use of prism lenses and vision therapy, we often see more appropriate emotional reactions, as well as a stimulation of language—both likely due to a reactivation of higher-level cortical pathways.[25]

The role of ambient prism lenses and vision therapy in a treatment plan

My experience shows that a visual management program incorporating ambient prism glasses and vision therapy typically results in rapid generalization of new skills, and permanent gains in performance and behavior. This is why I believe that no treatment program for autism, developmental delays, or learning disabilities can be complete unless it addresses and corrects the visual dysfunction that underlies so many learning and behavior problems. When we correct visual deficits, we facilitate all future learning, and powerfully enhance the ability of our patients to maintain and generalize the skills they acquire.

Moreover, while behavior modification is helping thousands of children with autism and other disabilities, there are limits to what education can achieve when sensory systems—and particularly vision, the dominant system in sighted humans—are compromised. We can use behavior modification to help improve poor eye contact, reduce "stims," and ameliorate academic and social problems, but these educational efforts will be vastly more effective if we learn *why* these problems are occurring and address their root causes. This is more rational than expecting individuals with autism or related disabilities to change behaviors that are, in reality, logical strategies for adapting to sensory disturbances. Modifying the behavior of an autistic individual who hand-flaps as a result of ambient visual deficits, for instance, is similar to telling a limping person with a rock in his shoe, "Walk without limping, and I'll give you ten dollars." You may succeed temporarily—but you will have far more success over the long term if you correct the problem that caused the altered behavior in the first place. This is why children who fail to respond to behavior modification before undergoing vision therapy frequently excel when we address their vision problems.

While yoked prism lenses play a vital role in this process, it is critical to realize that prism lenses are only a first step in a program of visual management. Generally, it takes months (or in some cases more than a year) for patients to obtain full, permanent benefits from prism lenses and vision therapy. For patients to achieve a "feeling of normalcy," this therapy must encompass both intersensory effects and intrasensory motor processing (see Chapter 5). My experience shows that the effects of ambient prism lenses, while initially remarkable, fade with time unless patients are given the opportunity to fully integrate and organize the perceptual changes brought about by wearing the lenses. In the next section, I will explain this process, beginning with the testing procedure and following through to selection of prism lenses and the planning of an appropriate therapy program that will result in long-term gains.

Key concepts of behavioral optometry and the use of prism lenses

Vision is our dominant sense. Its effects on human behavior, emotion, and performance are pervasive.

Central nervous system disorders are associated with dysfunctions of eye movements.

Visual resilience is directly proportional to the efficiency of eye movements and depth perception.

The symptoms we observe and measure when we evaluate a patient for visual deficits are not the problem, but rather the solution that the patient has devised in order to maintain a steady state.

In working with children with autism or other disabilities, we must evaluate the human organism as a whole, rather than evaluating the eyeball in isolation.

The goal of treatment is to view each individual's performance and determine how it can be raised to a higher level of performance, rather than to compare a patient's performance to that of the population as a whole.

What can be learned by experience can be changed by experience. Ambient vision is a dynamic process, and change and improvement can occur at any stage in life.

The major function of the nervous system is to direct the muscular system of the organism. Effective visual management requires an understanding of the neural underpinnings of ocular movement, body movement, posture, and behavior.

Prism lenses alter a patient's perceived reality. The feedback provided by this perceptual distortion allows the neuromotor system to reorganize visual processing. In time and with training, this reorganization becomes permanent. In short, vision therapy is the process of establishing order from disorder in visual processing, to allow a person to perform at a higher level.

The most effective vision therapy occurs when we recognize the perceptual style of each patient and understand that adaptation and performance are not homogeneous but heterogeneous. In other words, we must treat the individual, not the findings.

Actions and emotions compete for the same energy. Thus, the *physiology* of visual processing cannot be separated from the *psychology* of behavior.

Notes

1 Riesen, A.H. (1975) "The sensory environment in growth and development." In A.H. Riesen (ed) *The Developmental Neuropsychology of Sensory Deprivation*. New York: Academic Press.

2 See, for example, Birnbaum, M.H., Koslowe, K. and Sanet, R. (1977) "Success in amblyopia therapy as a function of age: A literature survey." *American Journal of Optometry and Physiological Optics 54*, 5, 269–275; Chryssanthou, G. (1974) "Orthoptic management of intermittent exotropia." *American Orthoptic Journal 24*, 69–72; and Birnbaum, M.H., Soden, R., and Cohen, A.H. (1999) "Efficacy of vision therapy for convergence insufficiency in an adult male population." *Journal of the American Optometric Association 70*, 4, 225–232.

3 Cited by Holland, K. (2002) in "The science of behavioural optometry." Monograph in recognition of the 10th anniversary of the founding of the British Association of Behavioural Optometrists.

4 Cohen, A., Lowe, S.E., Steele, G.T., Suchoff, I.B., Gottlieb, D.D. and Trevorrow, T.L. (2003) "The effectiveness of vision therapy in improving visual function." Position paper of the American Optometric Association.

5 Scharre, J.E. and Creedon, M.P. (1992) "Assessment of visual function in autistic children." *Optometry and Vision Science 69*, 6, 433–439.

6 Denis, D., Burillon, C., Livet, M.O. and Burguiere, O. (1997) "Ophthalmologic signs in children with autism." *Journal Francais d'Ophtalmologie 20*, 2, 103–110.

7 Kaplan, M., Rimland, B. and Edelson, S.M. (1999) "Strabismus in autism spectrum disorder." *Focus on Autism and Other Development Disabilities 14*, 2, 101–105.

8 Cited in "A Wisconsin blueprint to improve the health of individuals with developmental disabilities—invitational conference report: Health disparities and developmental disabilities in Wisconsin." Waisman Center, University of Wisconsin-Madison, February 2003.

9   Van Splunder, J., Stilma, J.S., Bernsen, R.M. and Evenhuis, H.M. (2004) "Prevalence of ocular diagnoses found on screening 1539 adults with intellectual disabilities." *Ophthalmology 111*, 8, 1457–1463.

10 Granet's findings were reported by Thomas D. Schram (2000) in "The eyes have it in attention disorder: Visual focus may be affecting mental focus," *Optometrists Network* (online), 20 April.

11 Grisham, J.D. (1986) "Computerized visual therapy—year one report." Palo Alto: American Institutes for Research. Cited in "The effectiveness of vision therapy in improving visual function." American Optometric Association, www.childrensvision.com.

12 Landry, R. and Bryson, S.E. (2004) "Impaired disengagement of attention in young children with autism." *Journal of Child Psychology and Psychiatry and Allied Disciplines 45*, 6, 1115–1122.

13 Cohen, A., Lowe, S.E., Steele, G.T., Suchoff, I.B., Gottlieb, D.D. and Trevorrow, T.L. (2003) "The effectiveness of vision therapy in improving visual function." Position paper of the American Optometric Association.

14 Wold, R.M., Pierce, J.R. and Keddington, J. (1978) "Effectiveness of optometric vision therapy." *Journal of the American Optometric Association 49,* 1047–1059.

15 *ibid.*

16 Cooper, J. and Duckman, R. (1978) "Convergence insufficiency: Incidence, diagnosis and treatment." *Journal of the American Optometric Association 49,* 673–680.

17 Flom, M.C. (1963) "Treatment of binocular anomalies of vision." In M.J. Hirsch and R.E. Wick (eds) *Vision of Children*. Philadelphia, PA: Clinton.

18 Ludlam, W.M. (1961) "Orthoptic treatment of strabismus." *American Journal of Optometry and Archives of the American Academy of Optometry 38,* 369–388.

19 Dolezal, H. (1982) *Living in a World Transformed: Perceptual and Performatory Adaptation to Visual Distortions.* New York: Academic Press.

20 Szentágothai, J. and Arbib, M.A. (1975) *Conceptual Models of Neural Organization.* Cambridge, MA: The MIT Press. (Also published as *Neurosciences Research Bulletin 12*, 3, 307–510 [1974]).

21 Flach, Frederic (1990) *Rickie,* New York: Fawcett Columbine.

22 Flach, F.F. and Kaplan, M. (1983) "Visual perceptual dysfunction in psychiatric patients." *Comprehensive Psychiatry 24*, 4, 304–311.

23 Gesell, A., Ilg, F.L., Bullis, G.E., Ilg, V. and Getman, G.N. (1970) *Vision: Its Development in Infant and Child.* Darien, CT: Hafner Publishing Company.

24 LeDoux, J. (1996) *The Emotional Brain: The Mysterious Underpinnings of Emotional Life.* New York: Touchstone Books.

25 The causes of the deficits we see in individuals with autism remain to be elucidated, but my experience indicates that to some degree these problems are genetically influenced. Often the parents of my autistic patients reveal that they have similar (although milder) visual problems, which may in part explain the elevated incidence of affective disorders, anxiety, and extreme shyness or social impairment seen in the families of children with autism. The same is true for other disabilities as well: the parents of patients with learning disabilities, emotional disorders, and developmental delays frequently exhibit perceptual styles resembling their children's, and experience lesser but similar problems in interacting with their environment.

Part II

The Kaplan Nonverbal Battery: Testing and Interpretation of Results

CHAPTER 3

Special Tests for Special Needs

The first step in correcting a patient's visual problems is to identify what those problems are. This is far easier said than done, of course, when your patient is autistic.

To facilitate the diagnosis of autistic patients, as well as other patients who resist standard testing, I use a novel series of testing procedures known as the Kaplan Nonverbal Battery. This battery is the outgrowth of decades of testing and treating "untestable" patients—a journey that began with one little girl named Amy.

Prior to treating children with autism, I performed many exams on learning-disabled children and never experienced any difficulty using standard optometric procedures. My first encounter with an autistic patient, around 1980, was an eye-opener. The child, Amy, was non-communicative and uncooperative. Upon entering my exam room, she screamed and threw a tantrum. She screamed even louder when I approached with my ophthalmoscope. In self-defense, I backed away, and decided instead to merely observe Amy's behavior. In such cases, I've always found that the best approach is to watch your patients, and allow them to teach you how to help them.

What I saw was a little girl who, though her eyes were wide open, was not using her vision to learn about her surroundings. For most of us, vision is the primary, dominant source of all information. Amy had fallen back upon input from secondary senses, touch and hearing.

It was obvious that if any exam took place with Amy, it would be far from standard. While an exam traditionally ends with a lens prescription, I decided to try something radical: I reversed the process, and began with a lens prescription.

I sent Amy's mother home with a pair of frames so Amy could practice wearing them, and we scheduled another visit. This time, Amy and her mother arrived with a copy of Amy's favorite *Sesame Street* tape. As she watched the tape, I observed her response to glasses containing yoked prisms with bases in varying directions. With each change in the direction of the prisms, she showed very different responses. With base-up yoked prisms, I observed increased visual attention, more erect posture, and head and body relaxation. With base-down yoked prisms, she tilted her head, gave the screen only intermittent attention, and tensed her body. I saw similar results when I asked Amy to stand on a balance beam while watching the video.

The clues I gained from these simple activities formed the basis of a visual management program that initiated dramatic changes in Amy's life—she went on to obtain language, and graduated from junior college at the age of 22—and led me to develop an entirely new approach toward testing "untestable" patients. Since meeting Amy those many years ago, I've continually refined my examination procedure. However, the underlying principle has changed little: *watching and wondering.* (I first heard this phrase used by noted optometrist Amiel Francke, who attributed it to behaviourist Nikolaas Tinbergen.)

Autistic, learning-disabled, and emotionally distressed children with developmental disabilities or emotional disorders show various degrees of disturbance of spatial function. They have a problem knowing where they are in space. More basically, they lack an awareness of their own physical parts and how they move. To varying degrees, they have shut down their visual processes, in an attempt to create some sense of order in a confusing world. They will clearly reveal all of these problems and more to clinicians, but not under the conditions of a traditional exam.

Traditional vs. performance-based evaluation

The limitations of standard testing are clear to anyone who deals with "untestable" patients. Typically, subjecting a nonverbal and non-cooperative patient (and particularly one with an autism spectrum disorder) to a traditional eye examination is an exercise in futility. Anyone with experience with autistic patients is well aware of their speech deficits, tactile defensiveness, hypersensitivity to light, and fear of medical offices.

Conventional testing pushes all of these buttons, and, in addition, it requires that patients follow directions that are often incomprehensible to a nonverbal individual. The result of such testing, all too often, is a frightened and uncooperative patient, meaningless test results, and a frustrating experience for all concerned. The same is true, in my experience, for many developmentally disabled or emotionally disturbed patients.

Moreover, conventional testing is a poor tool for detecting the visual problems that affect autistic, developmentally disabled, or emotionally disturbed patients. Most of these patients have adequate visual acuity, but experience difficulty in locating and identifying visual cues, as well as in integrating visual and other stimuli. Testing them for central processing in isolation will rarely lead to an understanding of their core problems, or to a workable visual management plan.

There are ways (which I'll describe later in this chapter) to modify the necessary tests for visual acuity and eye health when working with autistic or other "untestable" patients. However, the clinician who seeks to understand a nonverbal patient cannot rely solely on standard procedures, which assess a patient's ability to see form but fail to reveal problems in orientation or spatial perception. Experience has proven to me that the only way to gain a clear picture of what is happening with a nonverbal patient is to view dynamic real-life performance, with the understanding that symptoms are not problems but rather a patient's solutions to problems. By observing how an individual reacts to his or her environment, we can identify these solutions—toe-walking, head-turning, self-stimulating behaviors, squinting, fidgeting, abnormal posture, etc.—and formulate a diagnosis by asking the simple question: *How did this individual come to this solution?* The answer will guide us both in selecting the appropriate ambient prism lenses, and in developing the most effective therapy program.

As neuropsychiatrist Kurt Goldstein wrote, "It is of primary interest that the appearance of symptoms depends on the method of examination." If we evaluate a person with autism or related disorders using static tests of focal vision, we learn virtually nothing. If we test the same person in action, we can clearly see the adaptations that individual is forced to make in response to visual impairments—and from that knowledge, we can determine exactly what those impairments are, and how to address them.

What performance testing reveals

The series of tests included in the Kaplan Nonverbal Battery place a range of demands on a patient's ability to use the visual system to process information. The purpose of testing is to observe a patient's performance, both before and after exposure to yoked prisms, in order to see how the individual's sensory-motor apparatus copes with systematic alteration. As the clinician conducts each test in the battery, the patient can be evaluated for constraints in visual ability that manifest themselves in three areas:

- *Posture:* How does the patient hold his or her head and body? Does the patient toe in or out when walking, or toe-walk, or lean forward? Does the patient tilt his or her head? Does the patient exhibit functional scoliosis?

- *Attention:* Does the patient pay attention to the task? If so, how long is that attention maintained? Does the patient attempt to shut down one form of sensory input in order to attend to another—for instance, by covering his or her ears while watching a video, to reduce auditory input?

- *Disposition:* Is the patient relaxed or tense? Does the patient exhibit "stims" such as rocking or hair-pulling, or show facial expressions indicative of high stress? Do the patient's vocalizations indicate relaxation or tension?

A child's reaction to the tasks in the Kaplan Nonverbal Battery will reveal where deficits exist in the ambient vision system, shed light on how severe these deficits are, and provide necessary information as to how they can be corrected. As noted in Chapter 1, ambient vision skills are required to answer two critical questions: *Where am I?* and *Where is it?* Performance testing can provide us with a vivid picture of how well our patients cope with each of these questions, using visual processes both in isolation and in conjunction with other sensory modalities.

The first question, *Where am I?*, can be answered correctly only by a patient who possesses an accurate body schema. Famed neurologist Macdonald Critchley described body schema as "the idea which an individual possesses as to the physical properties of his own anatomy and which he carries over into the imagery of his self." Body schema involves visual, tactile, and labyrinthine components and is not inborn, but develops slowly as a child grows, always "tagging along" to some extent. An inability to create a valid corporeal schema will evidence itself in altered posture (head tilts, body warps, toeing in or toeing out), and in "stims" or self-injury, which often are a patient's way of creating body awareness. It is also the reason why some children are in constant motion: individuals unable to establish corporeal awareness through vision will substitute tactile information, which requires excessive movement.

Answering the second question, *Where is it?*, requires selective visual attention. Clinicians familiar with autistic individuals know that they display a fetish for numbers and letters, as well as spinning objects and running water. Higher visual development, in contrast, involves smooth eye movements and visual search patterns. The autistic pattern is marked by *static* attention, which is unsustainable, where the latter involves *dynamic* attention and is sustainable. Dynamic attention requires a concentration of internal energy, and patients who cannot coordinate their eyes are unable to achieve this level of concentration. Deficits in dynamic attention will clearly reveal themselves in tasks such as catching a suspended ball, which requires ongoing awareness of posture, visual motor coordination, and active organizing of time and space.

Using performance-based testing, the examiner is also able to evaluate the patient's response to tasks that require orchestration of the motor/ sensory complex. As optometrist Elliot Forrest notes, "Adaptation is a biological mechanism. Its purpose is to preserve equilibrium to counteract the effect of the stressor, and to minimize and delineate these effects to the smallest area capable of meeting the requirements of the situation." For some patients overwhelmed by conflicting sensory data, this will mean closing down several sensory channels—for instance, refusing to watch a video when the sound is on. For others, exposure to multisensory stimuli will cause signs of tension such as increased rocking, groin-touching, hair-pulling, or facial stress.

In addition, the Kaplan Nonverbal Battery will reveal clues about a patient's perceptual style. From a patient's reactions to the tasks, the clinician can learn whether the patient fights to process visual information, struggling to accomplish tasks despite repeated failure, or flees from processing visual stimuli by withdrawing or acting out. The tests also reveal which of the two primary styles of perception a patient uses: focal, or global. A patient who relies more on focal vision hones in on form and details, using eye fixations. A patient with a global perceptual style relies more on scanning the larger environment, using a repetitive sequence of saccades or scanpaths that allow the person to view the sub-features of a particular scene. The former type of patient views the trees, while the latter views the forest—and knowing which style a patient uses is crucial to selecting lenses and planning therapy.

When evaluating a patient's responses to tasks in the Kaplan Nonverbal Battery, it is important to recognize that the focus of this evaluation differs from that of standard testing, which is designed to compare individuals to the population as a whole. Instead, the Kaplan Nonverbal Battery is designed to determine if we can raise each individual's abilities in comparison with that person's own baseline performance. In general, if a clinician can observe changes in movement, attention, and motivation in response to ambient prism lenses, then therapy is likely to be highly beneficial.

Setting the stage: control, motivation, and preparation

A clinician's office can be a scary place, especially for an autistic child. Many autistic children seek a familiar daily routine, and do not like to venture into new places. Moreover, many are overly sensitive to lights, colors, smells, and sounds. Some are afraid of the dark. Most have been poked, prodded, and subjected to frightening and incomprehensible tests for many years, and have learned to fear medical professionals.

To reach these patients, the clinician must start off on the right foot. I begin by bringing new patients directly into my training room, which is filled with interesting toys, rather than taking them to an examining room with its intimidating instruments. In the therapy room, I allow them to explore their surroundings and handle any objects that draw their attention. I keep distracting sounds to a minimum, and no one in my office wears strong scents. Above all, I allow my patients to set the pace.

I'm often reminded, while waiting for my patients to find their comfort zone, of a story Gene Wilder once told about his first on-set acting experience. Wilder was very nervous, and when the director said, "Action!," Wilder immediately began blurting out his lines. After yelling "Cut!" the director gently explained, "Gene, you don't have to start talking the second I say 'Action.' Wait until you feel ready." Wilder said this advice made him feel so comfortable that he delivered a performance that earned him an Oscar nomination.

What is true for a nervous actor is even more true for the tense and frightened patients we ask to perform in a doctor's office. Given the chance, these patients will reveal their strengths and weaknesses—but only when they are fully ready. Moreover, clinicians can use this "getting acquainted" phase to learn a great deal about what makes patients tick (see "Pre-test evaluation" in a later section of this chapter).

One ten-year-old autistic boy, upon entering my training room before testing, started moving around the room to inspect his new environment. As his eyes caught hold of himself in the full-length mirror, his arms went up and he started to flap his hands. His problem, I knew immediately, involved an inability to pay attention to "self" and "space" at the same time. His solution: flapping his hands, to inform his brain that he had a body.

Casually, I walked over to him and placed a beanbag on his head, giving him immediate feedback as to where his body was in space. That extra bit of information about his orientation freed him from the need to continually "find" himself, and he responded by lowering his arms to his sides and standing normally.

Once testing begins, I continue to allow patients a great deal of flexibility in determining what they will and will not tolerate, an approach that proves very effective. For instance, not long ago, a colleague referred a 13-year-old with emotional problems. When I initially saw the girl, she yelled angrily, "I don't want to do this!" I responded by simply saying, "No problem—you don't have to." Surprised at being given control of the situation, she instantly responded, "No—I want to do it!" I then put her through the type of evaluation that I typically conduct with patients who are autistic, and she cooperated beautifully. Her mother remarked later, "That's the first time she's been in a doctor's office that we didn't have to put her in restraints."

An equally important key to a successful evaluation is motivation. Autistic and other developmentally disabled children typically have no idea why we're performing a vision evaluation, so it is no surprise that they often resist. To recruit them as allies, we must catch their attention by proving to them that vision therapy will make a positive difference in their world. That's why I typically move quickly to a ball-catching task, as soon as I've determined which ambient prism lenses are likely to work for a child. A child who's never been able to catch a ball successfully, and discovers that ambient prism lenses make this task easy, usually becomes a much more willing and active participant in both testing and therapy.

Another necessary step in creating the environment for successful testing is preparation, particularly in the case of autistic patients. Because individuals with autism exhibit extreme tactile defensiveness and resistance to new activities, the act of wearing glasses is highly stressful for many of them. To prepare them for the use of ambient prism lenses in my office, I ask their parents to obtain a pair of frames (with no lenses) several weeks before the exam, so the children can become accustomed to wearing glasses.

A note about history-taking

Almost all doctors take a history before beginning an evaluation, but I stopped doing this many years ago. Instead, I ask caretakers to fill out a history, but I explain that I will not refer to it until after my exam. I tell them, "I will predict your child's performance, behavior, and developmental history based on what I learn during my evaluation. If my description of your child's performance and behaviors matches your observations, then you will know that you're in the right pew."

Over the years, my experience has revealed the wisdom of Arnold Gesell's words, "To know the child, you must know the nature of his vision, and to know the nature of his vision, you must know the child." Translated into clinical practice, this means that once I know a child as a result of my evaluation, I can predict his or her behavior and performance—and once I evaluate an adult, I can reconstruct his or her development as a child.

A doctor who takes a history prior to performing an evaluation is focusing on a patient's structural and functional maladjustments, in order to predict the measurements and observations that he or she can expect during an exam. I take the opposite approach, believing that the symptoms a patient exhibits during an exam are the patient's solutions to maladjustment, and that these symptoms are clues that will point me to an understanding of the patient's underlying problems. In explaining this approach, I like to describe a logic class I once took, taught by a professor who also worked as a police detective. For our final exam in the class, our professor did not require us to answer abstract questions about logic. Rather, he presented us with the real-life facts of a crime, and asked us to use logical methods to uncover the identity of the criminal. Similarly, I use real-life observations of my patients to determine the identity of the "culprits" causing their visual dysfunctions. Those observations come from the Kaplan Nonverbal Battery, described below.

The Kaplan Nonverbal Battery

The tasks in the Kaplan Nonverbal Battery are arranged logically in a hierarchy that allows an observer to see how the child deals with increasing demands on the visual system. The initial tasks focus on visual perception in isolation, while succeeding tasks require the patient to coordinate visual, vestibular, proprioceptive, auditory, and gravitational input.

In each step, the clinician assesses the patient's posture, attention, and disposition in response to a visual demand, both before and after applying ambient prism lenses. To codify the results, I recommend using a scoring sheet (see sample provided at the end of this chapter).

Pre-test evaluation

You will be able to pick up many clues before formal testing begins, simply by observing your patients when they arrive. The vision problems of developmentally disabled children, and autistic children in particular, will manifest themselves in a variety of ways. Many patients will toe-walk, toe in, or touch the walls when they walk. These patients are unable to handle both self and space simultaneously. They will flap their hands to achieve balance, run their hands along the wall for tactile guidance, or toe in for orientation. They will walk on their toes because they do not trust themselves in space, and thus try to hold onto the ground for as long as possible. They often take shorter steps, which is also an attempt to maintain contact with the ground. Rather than sitting smoothly, some will need to feel for the chair and will sit awkwardly.

While many parents believe these behaviors are impervious to treatment, they actually are highly amenable to change. For instance, during my evaluation of a ten-year-old girl from Toronto, it became clear that she was a chronic toe-walker. Her heels touched the ground only when she stopped walking. I asked her mother, "Would you like to see your daughter walk with her heels touching the ground?" "Oh!" she exclaimed. "Yes—she always looks so awkward as she walks about." I placed ambient prism lenses on the girl's eyes, and she immediately began walking normally, landing on her heels and pushing off on her toes. Like this girl, the majority of toe-walkers have a spatial problem, and about 75 percent of the time ambient prism lenses will lead to an immediate change.

Your initial observation can also reveal signs of the functional scoliosis that often occurs in response to visual problems. This is important, because this problem can frequently be reversed with therapy. For instance, one 16-year-old learning-disabled patient I evaluated had a 20 percent curvature, and after identifying his vision problems, I told his parents that visual management could help resolve not only his problems with reading and sports, but also his spinal curvature. The mother clearly thought I was crazy, but the father said, "Let's give it a chance." Six weeks later, the orthopedic surgeon who'd previously recommended surgery measured the curvature, and found that it had gone from 20 percent to 12 percent, and that surgery was no longer needed.

Such cases illustrate the fact that a surprising number of the conditions that medical professionals believe are structural (and therefore not correctable) are in reality functional (and thus correctable) reactions to perceptual problems. And, to return to the topic at hand, they illustrate the importance of my primary rule of testing: *watch the patient, and you will discover the diagnosis.*

Once your patient is relaxed and ready to participate in testing, you can begin your formal evaluation. Here are the tasks, in order, that make up the Kaplan Nonverbal Battery:

Task 1: Video viewing

For this task, two chairs are positioned side by side, 4 or 5 feet in front of a 19-inch color TV monitor. One chair is for the patient, and the other for the parent or caretaker. The chair height must be low enough to allow the patient to place his or her feet flat on the floor. Parents are asked not to give any directions to the child, such as "Sit up straight," because it is important to observe the child's natural head and body posture.

Parents or caretakers are instructed to bring along one of the patient's favorite videos. For the first test, the clinician inserts the video, and observes the child's behavior before and after ambient prism lenses are applied. It is important to take very detailed notes, and I also recommend videotaping each session so it will be possible to review the visit later as an observer rather than as a participant. Among the factors to evaluate:

- Does the patient pay attention to the video? Is that attention brief or sustained? Is the patient attending to both visual and auditory input?
- Does the patient tilt his or her head while watching, or watch out of the corner of one eye?
- Does the patient exhibit stims while watching the video?
- Is he or she relaxed or tense?
- Does the patient exhibit strabismus/exotropia/esotropia?

Over 20 years, I have seen every possible variation of television watching. Some patients sit up straight while facing the screen. Others sit to the side or tilt their head sideways, avoiding binocular vision because their eyes cannot efficiently fixate on the same point. Some patients sit for only a short time, and then get up to touch the screen or play with the dials. Many engage in repetitive, self-stimulatory behaviors, commonly rocking side-to-side (using gravity to enhance their body awareness) or front-to-back (in an attempt to achieve depth perception). Some wrap their feet around the chair, sit on their hands, or grip the chair arms tightly, signaling that they cannot attend simultaneously to body sense and visual demands.

Often, the type of video the child prefers can be as instructive as the child's behavior. For instance, one of my patients chose to watch a tape of the Miss America pageant over and over, while another preferred tapes of the Weather Channel and a still another would only watch the credits of shows. Sometimes children will be comfortable watching certain sections of a video, but cover their ears, scream, or turn their eyes away during other sections. Such behaviors provide valuable insights into the type and amount of visual and sensory input a patient is capable of handling.

Once the clinician formulates an accurate idea of the patient's level of performance on this task, it is time to move to the next stage: determining which ambient prism lenses will successfully alter this performance. For this purpose, I use a set of standard optical frames in two sizes (for children and adults), color-coded so that it is easy to identify the types of yoked prisms: base-up, base-down, base-right, or base-left. (The types and effects of ambient prism lenses, and how to determine which are most likely to be effective for an individual patient, are discussed in Chapter 4.)

Typically, it makes sense to begin with the lenses most likely to precipitate a change that will be observable to the clinician, to the child's parent, and, most importantly, to the child. As each set of ambient prism lenses is applied, the clinician observes for changes in posture, attention, and disposition.

No two children are alike, but most children will clearly signal when a pair of lenses creates a significant change. One of my patients, for example, watched the television while poking one finger up his nostril, higher and higher. When I applied the correct ambient lenses, he removed his finger from his nose. When I gave him a second pair, with prisms in the opposite directions, up went the finger again. Another patient, a large and imposing autistic young man, maintained a constant, rhythmic running of his fingers through his hair, until I found the lenses that relieved his stress. With these lenses in place, he sat calmly and held his hands at rest, quietly watching the video.

Some children will reveal that a particular set of lenses is effective by exhibiting marked changes in attention. One autistic boy, for instance, listened to the sound of the video but turned his head away to avoid watching it. Given the correct pair of ambient prism lenses, he was able to process both visual and auditory input without becoming overwhelmed. In other patients, a response to lenses will be signaled by reductions or escalations in rocking, hair-pulling, groin-touching, leg movement, self-injurious behaviors, vocalizations, laughing, or facial grimacing.

Task 2: Video viewing with balance board

Task 1 evaluates vision in relative isolation, requiring only eye movements and not visually guided actions. Task 2 is a greater challenge, because it requires integration of the visual, proprioceptive, and gravitational systems.

This task is performed in the same room used for Task 1. This time, the patient is asked to stand on a balance board (16 inches by 16 inches, with a 3-inch by 2-inch fulcrum) while watching the same video used in Task 1. The child's responses will tell the clinician, on a "micro" level, how well the child can handle multisensory experiences in everyday life.

Experience has taught me to modify this procedure when a patient displays severe problems in orientation. For instance, if the child is so disoriented that the caretaker needs to hold his or her hand until the lenses are in place, I will begin with the patient seated on the balance board. Once the patient gains confidence, we can then switch to the standing position.

Again, the patient's reactions are tested both with and without ambient prism lenses. The clinician looks for changes in posture, attention, and disposition, as well as assessing the child's level of performance (can the child successfully balance while watching the video? How skillfully? For how long?) during the no-lenses and lenses conditions. When the right lenses are applied, the change between the no-lens and lens conditions should be readily detectable.

Task 3: Ball play

This task again ups the ante, by requiring a patient to exhibit visual-motor coordination, visual spatial judgment (timing), and intersensory coordination of localization. To catch a ball successfully, an individual must correlate the internal model of time and the external model of space. Any difficulty in making this temporal/spatial match will result in poor performance, a feeling of apprehension, and eventually a reduction in attention as the individual becomes frustrated by continual failure.

For this activity, the clinician will need a plastic baseball tethered to a string and set at chest level. When body schema is a severe problem, the patient can initially perform this task while seated, reducing the need for intersensory coordination. If a patient's deficits are so severe that catching the ball is impossible, switching from a ball to a balloon will slow the speed and allow the patient more time.

During this task, the clinician notes how well the patient attends to the ball, whether the individual moves toward the ball or attempts to dodge it, and whether the individual catches the ball itself or the string—all clues that can point to specific visual deficits. For example, one ten-year-old autistic girl who held her head constantly tilted displayed a "flight reaction" when the ball on the string was thrown in her direction. When I placed the correct ambient lenses on her, she stood her ground and reached out to catch the ball. The diagnosis: convergence insufficiency, a mismatch between where she perceived objects and where they actually existed. Her problem was a severe deficit in spatial perception, and her solution, in order to survive, was avoidance.

Once a clinician has a good idea of the patient's level of performance in this task, the task is repeated with the lenses that proved most beneficial during the earlier tasks. In most cases, patients will experience an immediate and dramatic improvement in performance. (This change is so marked that one response I frequently hear from verbal patients is, "What happened—did you throw the ball slower?") In addition to confirming the correct selection of ambient prism lenses, this change will motivate the patient to continue with testing and vision therapy.

The ball task also provides an excellent opportunity to give parents some first-hand insight into how disabling their children's visual deficits are, and how beneficial vision therapy can be. As parents observe the changes in their children, they typically ask, "What are these lenses? How do they work?" I find it easier to show them than to tell them.

Most of the parents of my patients have mild or moderate visual impairments themselves, but aren't aware of these problems. Often, when I throw a ball toward them, they exhibit some version of the symptoms their child has displayed. They quickly apologize, saying, "I haven't played in a long time," or, "I never really played ball." However, when I place the correct ambient prism lenses on the parents, and their ability immediately improves, they become quite excited. Like their children, they do not consciously feel the changes in their visual-motor behavior, but they can easily tell that the glasses are causing a significant difference.

Sometimes, however, the parents are experts at ball catching, without the help of ambient prism lenses. In these cases, I take a different tack. "In your child's case," I tell them, "I made them better; however, in your case, I will cause you to perform poorly." The next time I throw the ball, I have the parents wear disruptive ambient prisms, which precipitate a time–space mismatch of eyes and hands. Immediately they become tense, and grow irritated by the difficulty in succeeding at a formerly simple task—and they better understand just how unfriendly the world can seem to a child with severe visual dysfunction.

Task 4: Seated pursuits / Task 5: Standing pursuits

For the first of these tasks, the patient is seated in a comfortable position with the feet touching the floor. The examiner is seated directly in front of the patient. The target can be a Bruce wand, a shiny ball, or a finger, but I use a puppet figure placed on the head of a lit flashlight. This catches the attention of pediatric patients, and also amuses and relaxes adults.

The clinician first asks the patient to keep his or her eyes on the lit puppet, which is moved in a circular pattern followed by direct movements through the cardinal meridian. The clinician watches for the following:

- Can the patient sustain eye movement?

- Are the movements jumpy (saccadic)?

- Does the child follow with eyes alone, eyes and head, or even the body?

- Does the child reach with a hand to grab the object, or direct the eyes by pointing?

When there is a total lack of eye movement, the clinician should change the target to a bell. This will show the examiner if auditory input can influence eye movement and, if so, to what extent. If neither the lit puppet nor the bell elicits movement, the clinician should ask the patient to point at the puppet. Often, the addition of proprioceptive feedback will cue eye movement.

The clinician then repeats the pursuit procedure, this time with the patient standing. Perceptual style and degree of eye movement dysfunction will dictate whether a child performs better while sitting or standing. In either condition, the clinician watches to see if the child holds his or her breath, becomes hyperactive, or totally avoids the stimulus. These behaviors raise concerns about the visual stability centers, which receive information regarding the motor outflow to the eye muscle (third, fourth, sixth cranial nerves). The ability to judge observed movements depends on the interplay of information from these centers, which are responsible for the voluntary control of eye movements.

In both conditions, seated and standing, the testing is repeated with ambient prism lenses. The response of a child in these conditions is very significant for prognosis. For example, if I can solicit improved eye movement with ambient prisms during this task while testing a nonverbal or verbally delayed child with pervasive developmental disorder, I can in good conscience tell the parents that in four to six months we will get language.

Task 6: Mirror balance on one foot

In this task, the patient is asked to balance on one foot in front of a mirror. This tests a patient's ability to coordinate sensory modalities, as well as providing the clinician with a clearer picture of the child's developmental level. By the age of five, according to the Gesell Battery of Child Development, children should be able to sustain balance on one foot for the count of ten while looking at themselves in a mirror. Those who cannot may have significant issues with body schema. Some patients have significant problems in orienting themselves during this task because they cannot coordinate visual and vestibular input. These patients may have problems such as vertigo, motion sickness, and fear of heights.

Over time, the clinician will discover that some children place great importance on viewing themselves in a mirror, while others avoid their reflected imagery at all costs. This is a matter of perceptual style, and will be highly relevant later in designing a therapy program.

This task is performed with the patient standing first on the right foot, and then on the left (or vice versa). In each of these conditions, the task is performed first without and then with the ambient prism lenses. In each instance, the clinician observes posture, attention, and disposition, and notes the patient's ability to sustain the posture, the amount of tilt, the position of hands and arms, and where visual attention is directed.

Task 7: Television balance on one foot

This task is similar to the previous one (mirror balance on one foot) except that the patient is asked to balance while watching a video on television. The results of this and the mirror task offer the clinician insight into whether the patient is field-dependent (attends to space) or field- independent (attends to self). This information can be used later to design an effective visual management program.

Six-year-old Jimmy, diagnosed as autistic, had no trouble with the television-viewing and balance board tasks. When I asked him to balance on one foot while looking at himself in the mirror, however, he could not maintain his balance. As I watched, I could see that he gazed not at the reflection of his face, but at his feet. When I asked him to watch television while standing on one foot, however, he had no difficulty. He also responded to base-up ambient prism lenses. All of these observations told me that he needed to "lock on" to spatial cues, indicating that his visual style was global and field-dependent. A child whose visual style is field-independent, in contrast, will watch his or her own reflection in the mirror, avoiding spatial cues.

Task 8: Balloon play

This procedure is performed standing, and requires a 10-inch balloon. The clinician demonstrates to the child how to hit the balloon up in the air, first with one hand and then with the other, while counting from one to ten. The activity is then repeated, this time using the ambient prism lenses that have proven most effective.

In this task, the patient's visual system is forced to interact with both general and specific motor skills. To succeed at the task, a patient must be able to use the hands alternately, track the balloon when it goes over his or her head, and maintain a limited range of body movement. Poor performers tend to lose the balloon when it goes over their heads, or have trouble hitting it accurately enough to make it rise above eye level. In addition, they often must move excessively to keep up with the balloon, because they tend to hit it sideways rather than up.

Task 9: Walk and sit

This task requires two chairs, placed 8 to 10 feet apart. The clinician asks the child to walk from one chair to the other and then sit down, without touching the chair with his or her hands. The task is then repeated with the child wearing disruptive yoked prisms, using a magnitude of 15–20 diopters. With base-down lenses, the child will typically knock over the chair. In the base-up condition, the child will come up short of the chair.

With base-right prisms, the child will sit left of the chair, and with base-left, he or she will sit to the right of the chair.

The use of disruptive lenses allows the clinician to discover how a patient reacts to having his or her world visually transformed in a dramatic way. Does the individual walk slowly, or rush? Does he or she go down on all fours, and crawl across the floor? Does the patient shuffle cautiously, or lift the feet? Does the patient show fear and rip off the glasses, or seem delighted by the need to reactivate previously "turned off" visual processes in order to understand this new visual world? All of these reactions will tell the clinician how to proceed when planning a visual management program.

One young girl who came to my office had developed autistic behaviors and lost her ability to speak after suffering seizures following a DPT (diphtheria, pertussis, tetanus) shot. We tried a series of nonverbal tasks during her evaluation, but nothing happened. Since I was having little luck directing her visual system, I decided to disrupt it instead. After I placed disruptive lenses on her, she stood up in front of the mirror and began to dance and talk. It was an exciting experience for me and her mother, and the girl later did very well during visual therapy.

A NOTE ABOUT HANDLING TACTILE DEFENSIVENESS

As you conduct the tests I've outlined, one problem you are likely to encounter in patients with learning differences, autism, or related problems is "tactile defensiveness"—an extreme sensitivity to touch, which can cause a patient to cry, withdraw, or even strike out when touched. Frequently, patients with tactile defensiveness will exhibit associated symptoms such as hyperactivity and distractibility. Patients who are tactilely defensive frequently resist wearing prism lenses, even when they discover that the glasses help them to see and perform better.

In reality, we all display tactile defensiveness. Envision a roach crawling up your arm; instinctively, you would react negatively and emotionally to this sensation. People with autism spectrum disorders or related disabilities, however, often react equally violently to stimuli that most people find innocuous, such as wearing a hat or a pair of glasses. In extreme cases of tactile defensiveness, it's not surprising to see an autistic child strip naked to avoid the unpleasant sensation of clothing. Autistic writer Temple Grandin, who suffers from severe tactile defensiveness, says that new underwear is a "scratchy horror," and that the petticoats she wore as a child were like "sandpaper scraping away at raw nerve endings."

In working with patients who react strongly to tactile stimuli, it is important to understand the cause of their problem—and one of these causes is poor visual processing. Arnold Gesell, in discussing the evolution of the human action system, wrote, "Human behavior is a convenient term for all the reactions of the organism which are mediated by the neuromotor system." The early human brain relied on tactile, olfactory and auditory systems to direct the neuromotor system's responses to stimuli and determine if a "fight" or "flight" response is needed. Over many centuries, we've evolved to depend increasingly on higher-level visual and auditory senses, which allow us to quickly inhibit and modulate our actions and emotional responses to stimuli.

Many children with autism or related disabilities, however, are locked into trusting touch, taste and smell for movement arousal for fight or flight. Lacking an accurate body schema, and dependent on lower-level sensory input to identify threats, they survive by over-reacting to stimuli that the rest of us can accurately and quickly dismiss with the aid of efficient visual processes.

When a patient displays tactile defensiveness, and associated hyperactivity and distractibility, a struggle over wearing the prism lenses is likely to occur. Red flags include head tilting, visual avoidance, hyperactive movements, and emotional outbursts in response to tasks. To make it easier for tactilely defensive patients to accept wearing glasses, I introduce the glasses in an environment in which the field of view allows for the least possible amount of eye movement (for instance, while the patient is seated and watching television). In my experience, 80 percent of patients will accept the lenses immediately under these conditions, while the other 20 percent will accept them more gradually. To a great degree, a patient's ability to accept the glasses varies according to age, intelligence, and efficiency of auditory processing. The important thing is to persist, even in the face of strong initial resistance, if you are confident that the glasses will help your patient.

Jennifer was five when I first evaluated her. She was nonverbal and exhibited autistic behaviors, hyperactivity, and tactile defensiveness. My testing showed that she performed best when wearing base-down ambient yoked prisms.

Getting Jennifer to wear the glasses, however, was a challenge. Even though she displayed improved balance and hand–eye coordination with the prism lenses on, she resisted the sensation of having glasses on her face.

I knew that in time Jennifer would grow to appreciate her new abilities, and accept the glasses—but I also knew that this wouldn't happen instantly. So I instructed her parents to let Jennifer set the pace. They took the glasses home and each hour they placed them on her, allowing her to remove them whenever she wished.

A month later, Jennifer's mother called me, very excited. Jennifer was now wearing the lenses full-time, and was much calmer, less hyperactive, and more responsive to instruction. What's more, she clearly recognized that the glasses were helping her: each night when she took the glasses off, she would place them in their case, close the case, and then kiss it goodnight.

GESELL DEVELOPMENTAL ASSESSMENT

After completing the Kaplan Nonverbal Battery, the clinician can use standardized tests in order to determine the age level of the patient's performance. I use the block play, "incomplete man," circus puzzle, form puzzle, and "copy form" subtests of the Gesell Developmental Assessment, as these are appropriate for nonverbal patients and can be very revealing.

For instance, one sign of the delay in the development of children with autism and related disabilities can be detected in the "copy forms" task. Very young children can recognize a diagonal line and distinguish it from a vertical or horizontal line, but they cannot copy the diagonal line correctly. Typically, children master this copying skill by the age of five. Many autistic children, however, cannot copy a diagonal line because they have problems in differentiality (the perception of space and the perception of form), and accurate visual perception of form is needed for representational drawing. The inability to master this skill has developmental repercussions that go far beyond drawing, even affecting such motor skills as walking up and down stairs.

At the conclusion of the Kaplan Nonverbal Battery, you will have an excellent idea as to whether or not your patient will benefit from vision therapy, based on the individual's response to ambient prism lenses and his or her ability to achieve a higher level of performance. Most individuals with autism will not exhibit smooth eye movements, but if you observe changes in movement, attention, and a motivation to track visually, these are all indicators of a positive prognosis.

During the battery, you also will have identified:

- visual perceptual disturbances

- visual memory loss

- depth perception deficiency

- abnormal blink rate

- balance and posture difficulties.

In addition, your observations will tell you if your patient's perceptual style is focal or global. This will aid you in creating a visual management plan that builds on your patient's strengths while moving toward addressing weaknesses, and it will offer insight into how your patient is likely to respond to different tasks. For example, a child with a low level of global organization will usually grow fatigued in the afternoon, may tend to get headaches when presented with visual demands, and is likely to exhibit motion sicknesses.

You will know, too, whether your patient is field-dependent or field-independent. This will tell you whether your therapy plan should initially address *orientation of self* or *organization of space*, and whether the ambient lenses you prescribe should enhance orientation or organization. In addition, you will know which type of rehabilitation, directive or disruptive, will have the greatest effect on your patient. These findings will provide you with all of the information you will need to design an effective therapy program.

At this point, a conventional visual evaluation should be performed if possible. As I've noted, this can be a challenge with nonverbal and "untestable" individuals, but there are ways to make the experience far less stressful for your patients.

Adapting the conventional visual evaluation for the "untestable" patient

A conventional evaluation is designed to identify central dysfunction, in which the subject can see but is experiencing difficulty in seeing fine details of an object. This evaluation assesses:

- ocular health—the organic condition of the eye and adnexa

- ocular alignment of the eyes—the presence or absence of any structural/muscular defect that interferes with single binocular vision

- refractive status—myopia, hyperopia, or astigmatism.

Ocular health

Nonverbal and "untestable" patients, like all other patients, need to be screened for organic conditions such as cataracts, tumors, glaucoma, lack of coordination, or lack of color vision. Typically, clinicians do this by:

1. *Shining a light into the eye of the subject to obtain the pupil's response to light.* When the clinician shines a penlight into either eye, the pupil size should constrict. When the clinician shines the light into the right eye while blocking the light from reaching the left eye (by placing a hand on the patient's nose), the clinician should observe a "consensual response"—that is, contraction should occur in the left pupil as well as the right. This activity is repeated with the other eye.

2. *Examining the cornea, conjunctiva, lids, and the adnexa of the eyes.*

3. *Performing an internal examination of the eye using direct and indirect ophthalmoscopy.*

I've heard many horror stories (and virtually no success stories) from parents whose nonverbal children have been subjected to a standard ophthalmoscopy examination. These children often are so overwhelmed by the bright light and the proximity of the clinician that they require restraints or sedation.

It is my experience that this process becomes much less stressful to the patient when the examiner understands the special needs of patients with autism, other developmental disabilities, or emotional disorders. These patients often have a powerful fear of the unknown, and have a problem with people intruding on their personal space. To overcome the apprehension of a nonverbal patient, I first shine the light on the patient's hand and ask the patient to touch it. This allows the individual to realize that the light is non-threatening. Next—and this is very important—I place the patient's hand on the instrument as I move in to view the eyes. This puts the individual in charge, and in control of the situation. Finally, I give the patient something to view that will hold his or her interest as I move into position. I have chosen television watching, which is attractive to most children as well as adults.

Refractive status

Conventional measurements of ocular motor alignment measure static fixations. However, because misalignment leads to excessive eye movements, I am more interested in the dynamics of eye movements than in a patient's static view of the world. Moreover, the typical approach of evaluating monocular visual acuity and then evaluating binocular acuity is too demanding a procedure for most patients with autism or other developmental disabilities. It is stressful to cover one eye, and in many patients (particularly children) this elicits a flight response. Therefore, initially I am only interested in binocular acuity. Additionally, most autistic individuals have a fetish for numbers and letters, which is a strong indication that their focal vision is generally intact and that deficits in seeing for identification rarely play a role in autism.

However, visual acuity is important, so I modify the procedure by asking the patient to match a figure (e.g., boat, heart, cross, star) projected on the wall with one of two or three figures on a card. During the task, I observe how much time it takes the patient to match the objects, whether the patient attends to the task or avoids it, and whether the patient answers without even looking at the object on the screen. If I can establish 20/40 vision using this assessment, I am satisfied that the child can meet the focal demands of the environment.

Refractive errors

Refractive errors include myopia, hyperopia, and astigmatism. There are both objective and subjective methods for determining refractive errors, but the latter are not useful with nonverbal patients because they usually require verbal feedback.

The objective method for investigation is retinoscopy (skiametry). In this evaluation, the patient views a target while the clinician observes the direction of movement of the reflected light illuminated on the retina. The clinician looks for a "with" motion or an "against" motion as the retinoscope light moves across the retina. When the motion disappears, this represents the correction of lens power that the patient requires in order to see clearly (plus lens for hyperopia, minus for myopia, and cylindrical power for astigmatism). In addition, a bright reflex indicates a higher degree of attention than a dull reflex. This physiological parameter is associated with the speed of problem-solving.

Nonverbal patients, and particularly those with autism spectrum disorders, often resist this procedure. To calm their fears, I allow them to hold the retinoscope, and I use a video as the target to encourage their attention. In almost every case, I am able to achieve sufficient compliance to perform the task.

Tests for verbal, high-functioning patients: the Van Orden Star, Keystone Skills, and 21-point battery

Three of the tests that are most helpful in diagnosing vision problems aren't included in the standard Kaplan Nonverbal Battery, because they require a patient to respond to verbal directions, and/or to perform a fairly complex task. These tests should be used when you are evaluating a patient with learning disabilities, a patient with Asperger Syndrome or high-functioning autism, or any other verbal, cooperative, and relatively capable child or adult.

The Van Orden Star offers the clinician a two-dimensional representation of how a patient views the three-dimensional world. The Appendix describes the procedure in depth, including illustrations. Briefly, a Correct-Eye-Scope with transilluminated back is used. The target is a translucent paper with two vertical columns of small shapes (heart, cross, diamond, etc.) on the left and right sides. One column is the reverse of the other—for instance, the circle appears in the top position of the left column, and in the bottom of the right column—and the center figure in each column is a cross.

The clinician asks the patient to look through the eyepiece at the screen, and asks, "How many columns of figures do you see?" If the patient can see both columns, and can see them both at the same time (rather than alternating between the left and right columns), the clinician then hands the patient two pencils—one for each hand—and asks the patient to place the pencil points on the center cross in each column and draw simultaneous lines, one toward the other, until the pencil points look as if they're touching in the middle of the page. The patient is then asked to place the pencil point on the corresponding figures on the top right and bottom left sides, and to draw simultaneous lines inward toward the center until the lines appear to touch. This is repeated with each corresponding figure. The expected result is that the two sides meet, forming an apex at the midline of the vertical plane.

To create a correct Van Orden Star pattern, a patient must rapidly and accurate interpret what is viewed, generate a correct motor response, and maintain attention throughout the task. An imperfect Van Orden Star can indicate a wide range of impairments that are detailed more fully in the Appendix. (For example, a Van Orden Star in which both apices are well formed but meet below the line indicates a relatively minor problem in binocular coordination. When the drawings end above the line but fail to meet in a definite apex, there is a far more severe problem in spatial organization, and an individual will exhibit more serious behavior problems.) Thus, the organization, symmetry and placement of the apex offer insight into a patient's perceptual style and diagnosis, and aid the clinician in selecting the correct yoked prism lenses.

The Keystone Visual Skills Tests are of course familiar to most optometrists, as is the standard 21-point battery, which is routinely used by clinicians. Again, these tests require verbal ability, and even some verbal patients will find them difficult or impossible to complete. However, these tests should be incorporated in your evaluation whenever appropriate.

PERCEPTUAL ANALYSIS SCORESHEET (I)

Patient's Name:_____ Date:_____ Age:_____

HAB = baseline performance (using lenses if patient has a previous prescription)
BU = base-up lenses
BD = base-down lenses
BR = base-right lenses
BL = base-left lenses

TELEVISION SEATED

	Head Posture	Body Posture	Visual Attention	Disposition
HAB	4 3 2 1 0	4 3 2 1 0	4 3 2 1 0	4 3 2 1 0
BU( )	4 3 2 1 0	4 3 2 1 0	4 3 2 1 0	4 3 2 1 0
BD( )	4 3 2 1 0	4 3 2 1 0	4 3 2 1 0	4 3 2 1 0
BR( )	4 3 2 1 0	4 3 2 1 0	4 3 2 1 0	4 3 2 1 0
BL( )	4 3 2 1 0	4 3 2 1 0	4 3 2 1 0	4 3 2 1 0

TELEVISION BALANCE BOARD

	Head Posture	Body Posture	Visual Attention	Disposition
HAB	4 3 2 1 0	4 3 2 1 0	4 3 2 1 0	4 3 2 1 0
BU( )	4 3 2 1 0	4 3 2 1 0	4 3 2 1 0	4 3 2 1 0
BD( )	4 3 2 1 0	4 3 2 1 0	4 3 2 1 0	4 3 2 1 0

BALL PLAY

	Movement/Posture	Attention	Disposition
HAB	4 3 2 1 0	4 3 2 1 0	4 3 2 1 0
( )	4 3 2 1 0	4 3 2 1 0	4 3 2 1 0

PURSUITS SEATED

	Movement/Posture	Attention	Disposition
HAB	4 3 2 1 0	4 3 2 1 0	4 3 2 1 0
( )	4 3 2 1 0	4 3 2 1 0	4 3 2 1 0

PURSUITS STANDING

	Movement/Posture	Attention	Disposition
HAB	4 3 2 1 0	4 3 2 1 0	4 3 2 1 0
( )	4 3 2 1 0	4 3 2 1 0	4 3 2 1 0

PERCEPTUAL ANALYSIS SCORESHEET (2)

Patient's Name:_____ Date:_____ Age:_____

HAB = baseline performance (using lenses if patient has a previous prescription)
BU = base-up lenses
BD = base-down lenses
BR = base-right lenses
BL = base-left lenses

MIRROR BALANCE ON ONE FOOT	Head Posture	Body Posture	Visual Attention	Disposition
HAB	4 3 2 1 0	4 3 2 1 0	4 3 2 1 0	4 3 2 1 0
HAB R	4 3 2 1 0	4 3 2 1 0	4 3 2 1 0	4 3 2 1 0
HAB L	4 3 2 1 0	4 3 2 1 0	4 3 2 1 0	4 3 2 1 0
( )	4 3 2 1 0	4 3 2 1 0	4 3 2 1 0	4 3 2 1 0
( )	4 3 2 1 0	4 3 2 1 0	4 3 2 1 0	4 3 2 1 0

TELEVISION BALANCE ON ONE FOOT	Head Posture	Body Posture	Visual Attention	Disposition
HAB R	4 3 2 1 0	4 3 2 1 0	4 3 2 1 0	4 3 2 1 0
HAB L	4 3 2 1 0	4 3 2 1 0	4 3 2 1 0	4 3 2 1 0
( )	4 3 2 1 0	4 3 2 1 0	4 3 2 1 0	4 3 2 1 0
( )	4 3 2 1 0	4 3 2 1 0	4 3 2 1 0	4 3 2 1 0

BALLOON PLAY	Movement	Attention	Disposition
HAB	4 3 2 1 0	4 3 2 1 0	4 3 2 1 0
( )	4 3 2 1 0	4 3 2 1 0	4 3 2 1 0
( )	4 3 2 1 0	4 3 2 1 0	4 3 2 1 0

WALK AND SIT	Movement/Psoture	Attention	Disposition
HAB R	4 3 2 1 0	4 3 2 1 0	4 3 2 1 0
HAB L	4 3 2 1 0	4 3 2 1 0	4 3 2 1 0
( )	4 3 2 1 0	4 3 2 1 0	4 3 2 1 0
( )	4 3 2 1 0	4 3 2 1 0	4 3 2 1 0

Once you complete both the Kaplan Nonverbal Battery and a conventional vision evaluation, the final step of testing is to review your findings with parents or caretakers. (More on this in Chapter 4.)

On rare occasions, you will discover that a patient is unlikely to benefit from immediate therapy. When there is a poor response to either facilitative or disruptive ambient lenses during the Nonverbal Battery, the prognosis is guarded. However, this does not mean that such patients should be dismissed outright as poor candidates for vision therapy.

If neither the patient nor the caretaker can detect any change during testing, I typically send the patient home with rotating yoked prisms and ask the caretaker to try prescribed directions of placement, or to alternate placements on different days, to see if some positive movement occurs. If the response is positive, I have the patient return for a re-evaluation. In other cases, based on posture or a strabismic condition, I will ask the caretaker to have the patient wear yoked prism lenses as directed for one month, and then return. What I find, in a number of these cases, is that a patient who is too stressed to respond to testing in the office will respond in the safety and security of a home setting.

> One six-year-old evaluated in my office exhibited esotropia. He was also nonverbal and very aggressive, and other professionals had advised his parents to have him institutionalized. In my office, he did not respond on any level to the testing procedure.
>
> In cases involving esotropia, my clinical experience is that base-down yoked prisms often elicit very positive changes. Thus, I suggested that the parents try these lenses at home.
>
> When they returned to my office a month later, the difference was remarkable. The boy cooperated with testing, and he actively enjoyed the ball play task. I prescribed a program of therapy, and six month later his eyes were straight and he had language. Experiences like these tell me to be persistent when a child's future is at stake.

Fortunately, in the vast majority of cases, your findings will clearly reveal that your patients have visual problems that can be effectively addressed by ambient prism lenses and vision therapy. In these cases, parents or caregivers should be encouraged to pursue therapy as quickly as possible, because the more quickly a vision problem is corrected, the more likely it is that a child (or even an adult) can overcome visual problems and become a more capable, communicative, socially adept, and happy individual.

CHAPTER 4

Analyzing Your Test Results: The Art and Science of Knowing Your Patient

The tests in the Kaplan Nonverbal Battery are simple to perform, but interpreting your results requires both clinical intuition and experience. With time and practice, you will find that you can "read" your patients and interpret their symptoms with a high degree of skill.

As in all clinical practice, this ability involves both art and science. The science begins with understanding the way in which yoked lenses alter your patients' view of the world, and—by extension—their performance.

The effects of prism lenses

One of the most effective tools for altering a patient's perception of the world is a pair of yoked prism lenses. In Chapter 2, I discussed the rationale for using these lenses, and this chapter will offer case studies and "clinical pearls" that illustrate the process of selecting the right lenses for each patient. First, however, a quick review of the function of ambient (yoked) prism lenses is in order.

To begin with, all yoked prisms—no matter what type—differ from single prisms, the lenses typically prescribed by ophthalmologists and optometrists, in these key ways:

1. Single-prism lenses are *orthoptic*—that is, they are designed to correct muscular defects of the eyes. Yoked prisms, in contrast, are designed to alter *neural* function. Single prisms affect muscular orientation, while yoked prisms affect neural organization.

2. Single-prism lenses address *focal* vision, while yoked prisms address *ambient* vision.

3. Single-prism lenses address a patient's ability to identify objects—the "What is it?" function. Yoked prisms address a patient's ability to organize space and create a coherent body schema—the "Where is it?" and "Where am I?" functions.

4. Single-prism lenses are typically worn for the rest of a person's life once they are prescribed, because these lenses are compensatory. Yoked prism lenses are used to change the neuromotor processing of the brain, and when rehabilitation occurs, they are no longer needed.

Each type of ambient prism lenses alters space in a specific way. Table 4.1 outlines the different types of yoked prism lenses, and the way in which each type affects a patient's perception of space and, as a result, the patient's performance.

Table 4.1 Different types of prism lenses and their effect

Prism type	Effect on perception and performance
Base-up	Base-up prisms affect rotation about the horizontal axis in space, rotating the visual level of attention to a lower, closer field of view. There is a corresponding effect on the vergence system, improving spatial organization, sense of timing, and awareness of depth.
Base-down	Base-down prisms affect rotation about the horizontal axis in space, rotating the visual level of attention higher and farther away. There is a corresponding effect on the vergence system, improving spatial organization, sense of timing, and awareness of depth.
Base-left	Base-left prisms rotate the energy input about the vertical axis, moving attention toward the right field of view. This affects orientation, influencing posture, transport, and vergence eye movements.
Base-right	Base-right prisms rotate the energy input about the vertical axis, moving attention toward the left field of view. This affects orientation, influencing posture, transport, and vergence eye movements.

Typically, you will want to select yoked prism lenses that facilitate perception, allowing a patient to see the world in a more coherent and understandable way. However, I occasionally find it far more effective to begin with disruptive yoked prism lenses, which actually make a patient see the world as more chaotic. By distorting the vision of a severely withdrawn patient in this way, I can force the person to quickly abandon old strategies for coping, and leave the individual with no option except to pay attention to the environment. To explain this in a slightly different way, when low-magnitude "facilitative" yoked prisms are used (typically 5 diopters or less for testing, and 1 to 3 diopters when prescribed for autism or developmental delays), the changes that result are unconscious, and proprioceptive changes precede visual changes. When high-magnitude "disruptive" yoked prisms are used (usually over 6 diopters, and typically 15–20 diopters), the changes are conscious and force an immediate reorganization of the neuromotor system to meet the newly transformed demands of environmental tasks. Some patients need a feather, in the form of facilitative lenses; others need a hammer, in the form of disruptive lenses.

In either case, the long-term goal is to create a more ordered perception of the environment. Training then allows the patient to consolidate this new world view, at which point improved visual skills will be permanent and the patient can be weaned from the glasses.

Other professionals often ask me, "Which yoked prism lenses work best for each type of patient?" When patients are verbal and high-functioning, the correct prescription can be determined based on the results of the Van Orden Star (see Chapter 3 and the Appendix), the Keystone Skills, and the standard 21-point analytical battery. In these cases, prescribing of yoked prisms is predicted by:

- The Keystone level of fusion and the changes in the ocular alignment on the lateral muscle balance test, as the patient switches attention from a far-point to a near-point target.

- The organization or lack of organization, and where the pattern of lines is directed, in the Van Orden Star conducted at near-point.

- Phorometric testing (phoria, duction, AC/A, accommodation).

However, when patients are unable to perform these tests—and the vast majority of my patients fall into this category—there is no universal formula for selecting the right lenses for a given symptom or a given patient. Instead, the clinician must make a choice by observing each patient's responses to different lenses during testing. With time, you will develop an instinct for selecting the right lenses. Even then, however, lens selection is a combination of experience and some trial and error.

The following case studies help to demonstrate how this process works in real life, by describing the responses of a number of patients to testing, and how these responses pointed me toward the correct selection of lenses.

John: A case study illustrating the effects of prism lenses on posture

John, a shy, non-confrontational seven-year-old, came to my office after a visit to an ophthalmologist who diagnosed him as a high-hyperope, anisometropic amblyope with best corrected acuity O.D. 20/60, O.S. 20/30. John's mother, concerned about additional symptoms including John's poor motor coordination and learning problems, sought a second opinion prior to ordering the lenses. Among my observations during John's visual perceptual consultation:

- John's performance in the Keystone Skills—which provide information about binocularity, ocular alignment, level of fusion, and depth perception at both far and near—revealed that his ocular alignment was compressed.

- Because John was verbal and capable of following instructions, I included the Van Orden Star (which is designed for far-point and modified in my battery for near-point) in my testing. This visual projection test, described in the previous chapter and in the Appendix, demonstrates a patient's eye–hand coordination, level of orientation, and organization of space. John was unable to perform on this test.

- Observing John's posture, I noticed that his head tilted left.

- Habitual visual acuity testing (without lenses) revealed right eye acuity of 20/30, left eye acuity of 20/40, and an acuity for both eyes of 20/30. My suspicion was that John's ophthalmologist had used an evaluation conducted while John was medicated as the basis for his prescription. Retinoscopy indicated low plus.

Clinical pearl: When seating a child in the examination chair, I ask the child to press the "up" button controlling the chair. If the child pushes the button and immediately becomes startled and removes his or her finger, as John did, I suspect balance problems due to impairments in orientation.

- During visual pursuit testing with John seated, I saw that when the pursuit movement required vergence, John used his eyes but tilted his head further left, and his eye movements became saccadic. When I repeated the task with John standing, I noted that his eye movements were developmentally immature. In this condition, John now tracked using his head, not his eyes. (The normal age at which children become able to move their eyes while holding their head still is five years.)

- Phorometric testing for alignment and vergence were unreliable. The red lens test indicated eye fusion at far and diplopia at near, alternating with suppression.

My observation during the Kaplan Nonverbal Battery more clearly revealed the nature and scope of John's impairments:

- During seated television viewing, John tilted his head left, and was very fidgety. John responded better to base-left than base-up prisms, telling me that to survive, he was forced to pay greater attention to self (body schema) than to space. With base-left prisms in place, his head straightened, his attention increased and his fidgety body movements decreased.

Clinical pearl: When a patient's head tilts left, the use of base-left or base-up yoked prisms is indicated. When the head tilts right, base-right or base-down is indicated.

- When I asked John to stand on the rocking board and watch television, he was fearful of stepping onto the board and needed his mother's help. Rather than moving, he held his body stiff with his arms bent. He was extremely tense, and he paid only intermittent attention to the television. With the yoked base-left prisms on, he relaxed, his arms went down, he rocked confidently, and he watched the television with a smile on his face.

- In the ball play task, John was tense. He showed poor attention to the ball, and failed to reach for it. As a result, the ball hit him in the face. With the yoked base-left prisms on, he relaxed and paid attention. When I threw the ball, he reached out and caught it.

- When I asked John to balance on one foot, he could not sustain his balance. With yoked base-left prisms on, he improved significantly but still had difficulty.

- When asked to perform the "copy forms" task on the Gesell Developmental Assessment, John tilted his head left, and his drawings were disorganized with round corners on the squares, rectangles, and triangles. (Developmentally, a child should be able to draw the corners of a square or rectangle at age four, the corners of a triangle at age five, and the corners of a diamond at age eight. Each skill places an increased demand on perceptual organization and eye–hand coordination.) When I placed the base-left prisms on John, he organized his drawings in a normal left-to-right sequence, made sharp edges, and held his head straight.

Describing my findings to John's parents, I explained that the tilting of his head, his fears of balance, his poor eye pursuits and his inability to catch a ball stemmed from functional, not structural, neuromotor interference with the teaming of his eyes and with his ability to organize and integrate the input from his senses. When we placed the prism lenses on John, I explained, it reduced the need for him to block the actions of his nervous system, and allowed sufficient "information flow" for him to know where his own body and other objects were.

Because of John's strong positive response to ambient yoked prisms, I could confidently give his parents a positive prognosis. I explained that we would start John with the base-left prism lenses, to stimulate an improved awareness of orientation and body schema. The visual training procedures John underwent would allow him to reorient his neuromotor complex to the new reality created by the prism lenses. Once John consolidated these gains, I told his parents, we would change him to base-up prism lenses, and use vision therapy to address his spatial awareness. Eventually, yoked prism lenses would no longer be necessary for John, although he would probably need standard glasses to address his focal acuity.

I outlined realistic goals for John: in three months, he would be able to ride a bike, and his asthenopic symptoms would be reduced. His social interaction, too, would markedly change. I also predicted that in six months, we would see positive changes in his academic performance. I cautioned John's parents, however, to expect some interesting times when their withdrawn, timid child reached out to experience the world around him. "John will start challenging you instead of being a passive wallflower," I warned them. "He will become belligerent."

All of these predictions came true, including the last one. John made remarkable progress in school, and mastered riding his bike. Three months after he started wearing the prism lenses and entered vision therapy, he also got into his first playground battle. Each week for some time afterward, John's mother complained that John was getting into scuffles, even giving one boy a bloody nose. I was quietly pleased, because my training in childhood development taught me that all normal developmental stages involve "acting out" as well as positive behavior changes. John's mother, however, although delighted at his dramatic improvements in other areas, was less than thrilled by his new reputation as a playground contender. After the third or fourth fist-fight, she said to me, "You don't understand, Dr. Kaplan. This is a parochial school, and you can't act that way!"

Amber and Martin: Two case studies illustrating the effects of prism lenses on toe-walking

Many autistic children and adults walk on their toes. In studying this behavior, I was influenced by orthopedist Edward Schwentker, who wrote that "toe walking has multiple etiologies ranging from idiosyncratic habit to profound neuromuscular disease... In dealing with this entity, the underlying pathophysiology for each case must be understood to ensure that the treatment is appropriate to the specific etiology." Schwentker noted that while we can sometimes identify the cause of toe-walking—for instance, in cerebral palsy—the etiology often is idiopathic (in other words, "We don't know").

As I worked with autistic children, I discovered that in most of the cases considered by doctors to be idiopathic, toe-walking was not a "hardware" problem but rather an adaptation to distorted perception—a "software" problem. My proof: in many cases, I could alter the behavior quickly and effectively, simply by applying prism lenses.

One two-and-a-half-year-old girl, Amber, was a case in point. Referred to my office a few months ago with a diagnosis of pervasive developmental disorder, Amber responded only to visual or tactile stimuli, although her hearing was normal. She had poor eye contact, tilted her head, and toe-walked.

In the course of testing Amber, I saw that her head tilted left during seated television watching. When I placed yoked base-up prisms on her face, she straightened her head but fought against wearing the glasses—a typical response of children with tactile defensiveness. After a few tries she relaxed and began to smile.

Asked to stand on the balance board while watching television, Amber initially needed help from her mother. With the base-up prisms on, she could stand alone, and her visual attention to the television increased. In the ball play task, I modified the procedure by asking Amber to sit rather than stand, and I used a 9-inch balloon rather than the small ball. With the prism lenses on, Amber reached for the balloon.

Clinical pearl: Individuals with delays in multiple sensory modalities are forced to departmentalize, and cannot use more than one modality at a time. When you detect this problem in patients, test them in a seated position so they do not need to deal with gravity.

Amber toe-walked more frequently when barefooted than when wearing shoes. I tested her bare-footed, placing disruptive yoked 20-diopter base-down prisms on her, and she proceeded to walk flat-footed. By altering her perception dramatically, and foiling the adaptations that previously worked well for her, I forced her to reorganize her neuromotor system. The yoked prisms caused her to shift her body position in relation to gravity, putting her back on her heels and leading to more secure balance. This told me clearly that her problem was functional, not structural.

I prescribed yoked base-up prisms and an office-centered visual training program, which Amber has followed for three months. She now walks with a normal gait, pushing off on her toes and landing on her heels. She responds well to receptive speech, and her verbal expression is increasing.

Martin, another patient of mine, also toe-walked, although he wasn't autistic. A bright and articulate nine-and-a-half-year-old, Martin had poor coordination, sensory problems (particularly hypersensitivity to sound), and poor motor planning. His mother, who'd read about our center on the Internet, brought Martin to me to see if his toe-walking could be corrected.

Martin's visual acuity was 20/80, corrected to 20/20 with glasses. He exhibited adequate fusion and alignment at far and near, but also showed evidence of unstable fixation. His Van Orden Star pattern was disorganized, and below the line.

Clinical pearl: A Van Orden Star pattern that is drawn below the line and is disorganized indicates a scanning pattern with excessive eye movement, and poor localization and organization of space. In these cases, base-up yoked prisms are indicated. When individuals draw apices above the line, base-down prisms are indicated.

Martin's eye pursuit movements while seated were saccadic and displayed fast alternation. When standing, he was unable to track. Both seated and standing, he responded positively to yoked base-up prisms. He exhibited poor resilience on vergence, inwardizing movements both far and near. He also had a low AC/A ratio, and limited accommodative flexibility. His attempts to make chalk circles showed problems with figure/ground perception. Visagraph recording of his eye movements during reading showed inefficient fixations and regressions and delayed word recognition, but Martin's score on reading with comprehension exceeded expectancy—all signs that he had problems in identifying *where* words were (an ambient vision function), not *what* they were (a focal vision function).

In the ball play task, Martin tried to move away when the ball came toward him. With the yoked base-up prisms, he reached out and caught it. But his mother was even more excited by Martin's reaction when I asked him to walk toward a mirror. Without prism lenses, he walked with his body forward, and stayed up on his toes. When I placed the glasses on him, he stood erect, and walked flat-footed.

Martin wore his lenses (minus lenses for acuity and yoked prisms for spatial organization) for a year, while undergoing a program of visual management. By the end of that time, he walked flat-footed with an erect posture, and was much happier and far more secure emotionally and socially. His hypersensitivity also disappeared.

The cases of Amber and Martin illustrate two points. One is that toe-walking often is a child's way of adapting to a misperceived world, rather than a structural defect, and thus can be corrected—and typically very quickly. The other is that in vision therapy, "one size doesn't fit all." The selection of lenses depends on the individual, because as the cases of Amber and Martin show, very disparate visual impairments can result in the same behavior.

In fact, Amber and Martin are somewhat unusual because most patients who toe-walk have a focal ("tunnel vision") perceptual style, and yoked base-down prisms typically work best in these cases. But Amber and Martin both exhibited signs of overcompensated global organization—an adaptation in which individuals who are "scanners" by nature overcompensates for visual defects by jumping to the other extreme, and developing tunnel vision. This causes them to pay less attention to their surroundings, and makes them unable to use spatial cues. For such individuals, toe-walking is a survival instinct—a response to their altered posture in reference to gravity, which in turn stems from their reliance on kinesthetic rather than visual cues. Base-up yoked prisms transform light in a way that stimulates these patients' spatial organization, increasing the amount of information they can receive from the ambient visual system. As a result, they increase their visual attention to their surroundings, reducing their need to substitute kinesthetic for visual information. The result: a sense of security, allowing them to walk flat-footed with confidence.

In short, toe-walking is often correctable with prism lenses and therapy, but there is no one right lens prescription for a toe-walker. The answer lies in each patient's adaptation to his or her perceptual style.

Vicki: A case study illustrating the effects of prism lenses on rocking

Many individuals with autism spectrum disorders, including very high-functioning children and adults with Asperger Syndrome, rock back-and-forth or side-to-side. Doctors typically label this as a self-stimulating behavior, but that definition—while true in a limited way—doesn't accurately explain the true purpose that rocking serves.

Typically, rocking is the survival response of a patient who is unable to answer either the question of "Where am I?" (indicating a problem of orientation), or the question of "Where is it?" (indicating a problem in organizing space). For the clinician, the *direction* in which a patient rocks is as important as the rocking itself. Blind musicians—Stevie Wonder, for instance—often rock in a side-to-side direction. These individuals do not suffer from impairments in spatial organization ("Where is it?"); rather, they have problems maintaining an erect posture in the absence of visual cues. Rocking from side-to-side provides them with the neuromotor information they need to maintain upright while sitting or standing. The same is true of many autism spectrum children, and also of non-disabled individuals asked to pursue a visual target while standing.

In the case of a child or adult who rocks front to back, there is a different need: the need to compensate for a lack of depth perception. I saw an interesting example of this during an evaluation of a girl named Vicki, diagnosed as autistic. When I explained to Vicki's father that she had difficulty with vergence awareness—causing a mismatch between where she aimed her eyes and where the object actually was—he said that he had a similar problem. "What do you do for a living?" I asked the man. He replied, "I'm a portrait artist." I asked him how he perceived depth in his subjects, and he demonstrated by putting one foot in front of the other and rocking back and forth. In order for him to perceive depth, he did exactly what children on the autism spectrum do: he measured the depth physically, because he couldn't do it with his eyes alone.

Clinical pearl: In addition to rocking forward and backward, children on the autism spectrum who have difficulty with convergence also tend to move their heads toward a target, and have difficulty releasing a beanbag when asked to throw it.

In Vicki's case, I prescribed 2-diopter yoked base-up prisms. Her problem was that the mismatch between "where" an object was and "where" she aimed her eyes required her to make excessive eye movements in order to center on the object. Yoked base-up prisms, by transforming the light reaching Vicki's eyes, signalled a change in the position of an object (for instance, a ball coming toward her), allowing the nervous system to respond more efficiently and reducing the number of eye movements Vicki needed to make.

When I treated Vicki with yoked prisms and vision therapy, the changes in her neural system allowed her to perceive depth and see her world three-dimensionally. As a result, she rarely rocks, is much less anxious and hyperactive, and exhibits much better visual attention and receptive listening.

Vicki's case is a classic illustration of the axiom that "vision stops action." If a child can't answer the questions "Where am I?" or "Where is everything else?" simply by looking, he or she will be forced to use other senses—vestibular, proprioceptive, touch—to answer these questions. All of those methods require action, which is why so many children with autism and related disorders are labeled as hyperactive, or as having self-stimulating behaviors. In reality, many are using motion to compensate for visual deficits. When we remediate those deficits, the most "hyper" children often become relaxed and calm for the first time in their lives.

Ira: A case study illustrating how prism lenses can remediate poor functioning due to structural problems

Many patients' symptoms—for instance, toe-walking—initially appear to stem from structural defects, but actually are functional adaptations to visual deficits. However, you will also see cases in which structural defects lead to impaired function. Even in these cases, where "hardware" rather than "software" is the root of the problem, the right prism lenses can create positive changes.

A few months ago, for example, I evaluated Ira, a seven-year-old diagnosed with ocular albinism. In this rare inherited condition, the skin and hair have normal or nearly-normal pigmentation but the eye has very little pigment, and the fovea does not develop normally. The routing of nerve fibers from the eye to the brain is atypical as well, with a larger-than-normal number of fibers crossing from each eye to the opposite side of the brain. These defects lead to drastically reduced acuity, abnormal nystagmus, strabismus, and sensitivity to bright light.

Ira exhibited all of these symptoms, including a horizontal pendular nystagmus. His best corrected visual acuity was 20/120 O.D. and O.S., and his near vision with bifocal correction was 0.8m O.U. at 10 cm. Without lenses, his visual acuity was 20/100 at distance, and 20/30 at near. His mother told me that Ira refused to wear his prescribed glasses, which were bifocals with plus spheres and minus cylinders and a high bifocal add. Retinoscopy findings were inconclusive, due to his poor visual attention.

Ira was very active, and loved playing soccer and basketball. It didn't surprise me that he'd picked two sports that use big balls, in order to compensate for his poor vision. Unlike many of my patients, whose primary difficulty lies in ambient vision, Ira had difficulty with focal vision as well, due to his foveal defects. He exhibited both pathological and non-pathological saccades.

In the television-watching task, Ira was hyperactive and highly stressed, and paid only fleeting attention to the video. I turned off the volume and his visual attention improved, showing that he paid more attention to auditory cues than to visual ones. When I tried 5-diopter base-up prisms, Ira's posture and his attention to the video improved significantly.

In the rocking board task, Ira feared getting onto the board and could not maintain his attention. His attention improved when I applied the base-up prisms, as did his balance. During the next task, ball play, he was much readier for the ball when wearing the base-up prisms.

I also asked Ira to perform two seated-pursuit tasks. In the first, I asked him to wear disruptive +4.00 lenses in each eye. By interfering with his focal vision and making it harder for him to identify objects, these lenses slowed his nystagmus movements. In the second task, I asked Ira to catch a ball while seated, wearing disruptive yoked prisms placed 20 base-up over the right eye and 20 base-down over the left, placed over anaglyph red and green lenses. This created the illusion of two balls, one higher than the other, one red and one green. Ira was agitated at the beginning of this activity but then relaxed, and when I removed the disruptive lenses and the anaglyph glasses, his nystagmus was much less noticeable. I retested his visual acuity, and found that both the letters on the eye chart and the objects in the room appeared more clear and well-defined to him. As often happens in testing, disrupting Ira's vision had given his neural system a jolt that immediately altered his perception of his environment.

While Ira's prognosis for visual improvement is guarded, due to his severe innate structural defects, his heightened response to ambient cues while wearing either facilitative or disruptive base-up prisms told me that vision therapy could help him. He is currently participating in a visual management program, and we expect to see positive changes in his visual attention and eye–hand coordination, as well as less hyperactivity.

My optimistic prediction for Ira is based on similar cases, including one involving an 18-year-old woman with a pathological nystagmus and a visual acuity of 20/80. Like Ira, this young woman exhibited both slow- and fast-phase nystagmus, and she was quite frustrated because she continually failed the test for her driver's license. Intervention with yoked base-up prisms and vision training slowed her nystagmus, and improved her acuity to 20/40+—and it also resulted in a successful driver's license test. Toward the end of her therapy, she told me, her boyfriend asked what was wrong with her eyes. "What do you mean?" she asked him. He replied, "They've stopped jumping."

As a clinician, you will see a variety of abnormal nystagmus patterns, and often—as in these cases—they will respond to therapy. In many cases, the nystagmus stems from central nervous system defects, and indicates a poorly organized perceptual style. In other cases, such as Ira's, the nystagmus is an adaptation to structural defects. In either case, an abnormal nystagmus interferes with perception, which requires some degree of continuous movement across the retinal image.

Many patients, like Ira, exhibit both slow- and fast-phase nystagmoid movements. Neuro-ophthalmologist Patrick Lavin, M.D., notes, "The slow phase is pathological and is responsible for the initiation and generation of the nystagmus, the fast (saccadic) is merely corrective, bringing the fovea back on target." The goal of therapy is to slow the nystagmus, keeping the fovea on target as long as possible.

Clinical pearl: Yoked base-up prisms stimulate convergence, reducing the fast phase of nystagmus and helping to stabilize the environment. Clinical experience shows that yoked base-up prisms are highly effective for patients with motion sickness, vertigo, and asthenopic symptoms of headache and stomach disorder, all of which are symptoms of the vestibular dysfunction typically associated with nystagmus.

Tony: A case study in the effects of prism lenses on attention

Our skill in communicating with others, our success in forming personal relationships, and our achievements in school and on the job—even our very survival—all depend to a great degree on our ability to focus our attention on what's important. Most of us can do this instinctively and easily, but for the person with ambient visual impairment, there is nothing simple about "just paying attention." Unable to isolate and focus on relevant stimuli, some people with visual problems are easily distracted by every sight and sound, while others "tunnel in" and become functionally blind or deaf to critical cues in their environment. In either case, the correct yoked prism lenses, combined with vision therapy, can improve patients' selective attention skills.

Tony, a four-year-old patient of mine, is a good example. Referred by his speech therapist, Tony had developed normally until the age of 18 months, but lost his speech and developed autistic symptoms following his DPT (diphtheria, pertussis, tetanus) vaccination. His mother asked me to address his severe learning and attention problems.

When Tony entered the examining room, he walked on his toes—a typical sign, as I noted earlier, of a tunneled perceptual style. This indicated either problems with orientation, indicating the need for base-right yoked prisms, or problems with spatial organization, indicating the need for base-down yoked prisms.

During the television task, Tony fidgeted constantly, paying only brief attention to the screen. When he did attend to the video, his eyes alternated in an esotropic pattern. He also tilted his head to the right, another clue pointing to a tunneled perceptual style, and when he stood, his left foot was usually placed forward. This told me to try yoked base-right or base-down prisms. When I tried both sets of lenses, the base-down prisms reduced Tony's hyperactivity and immediately improved his attention.

When I asked Tony to stand on the rocking board while watching TV, he again performed better with the base-down prisms, relaxing and paying more attention to the video. The ball play task, which I did next, was particularly interesting. Initially, Tony failed to respond to a thrown ball, either with or without the base-down yoked prisms. This indicated that he did not pay attention to distant cues, because his world was two-dimensional rather than three-dimensional. I switched to a balloon, and when wearing the base-down prisms, Tony reached out and caught the balloon.

After he became comfortable, because of the balloon's size and slower speed, I switched back to the ball. This time, he reached out and hit the ball away—a defensive reaction caused by his new-found ability to perceive depth.

In the seated pursuits task, Tony paid more attention to the bell than to the lit finger puppet, a clue that he relied extensively on auditory cues to compensate for his visual attention deficits. His movements were smooth, but he could not sustain his attention.

When I probed Tony's reaction to disruptive yoked base-down prisms, he was startled and tried to rip the glasses off. His mother and I held his hands, and after a few minutes, he relaxed. Continuing to hold his hands, we walked him around the room, releasing him as he grew accustomed to the glasses. After a few minutes, Tony started experimenting with his gait. When I tried to take the lenses off, he reached out to take them back. I changed the position of the lenses to base-up, and he experimented again. I rotated the lenses back to base-down, and he walked with his feet flat on the floor. By dramatically altering his perception, the disruptive lenses had caused an instantaneous reaction by his neural system.

Tony's quick and positive responses to facilitative and disruptive prisms—which amazed both his parents and the Applied Behavioral Analysis instructor who came with them—made him an excellent candidate for vision therapy. As I predicted to Tony's parents at our first meeting, his visual attention improved markedly within two to four weeks of yoked prism use and therapy, and his receptive listening greatly improved within a month. Within a few more months, he developed useful language.[2]

Sara: A case study illustrating the effects of prism lenses on a child with a history of physical and emotional trauma

At eight months of age, Sara suffered a terrible fall and sustained a head injury that left her with gross and fine motor delays, speech delays, and balance problems. Her parents brought her to my office when she reached elementary-school age, because her school complained about her aggression, poor social skills, and difficulty in following directions. Her mother told me, "Sara is easily distracted, and works best in small areas where there aren't a lot of visual stimuli. Her teachers have to constantly remind her to do her work. Sometimes when she doesn't want to do tasks, she becomes very non-compliant, and hits or kicks or scratches." Sara's diagnosis was ataxia—that is, difficulty in coordinating voluntary muscle movements—which can stem from any of several disorders of the nervous system.

Sara's physical exam revealed that she had limited verbal skills, and sometimes drooled. She toed in, sometimes with the left and sometimes with the right foot. Her retinoscopy result was low plus.

During the video-watching task, Sara paid attention to auditory but not visual cues. Her head tilted left, and her ocular alignment showed a left exotropia. She had poor visual attention, and was highly stressed during this simple task. I tried yoked base-left prisms, which improved her head posture, visual attention, and disposition, and then yoked base-up prisms, which produced even better results.

In the balance board task, Sara did not improve when wearing the prisms. During seated pursuits, she exhibited poor eye movements and could not pay attention to the tasks. She improved noticeably with the base-left prisms on, especially when tracking the bell I used as a target. In the ball play task, which I performed with Sara seated, she did not attempt to reach for the ball, and she was fearful and unable to pay attention. When I placed the yoked base-left prisms on her, and used a 9-inch balloon as a target, she began paying attention, and started reaching for the balloon.

Next, I observed Sara as she walked around the room. When I placed disruptive 20-diopter base-down yoked prisms on her, she immediately began walking flat-footed.

Sitting across from Sara, I asked her to touch my hands with hers. She had no problem with this task. She also had no problem raising her feet while seated. However, she did have trouble raising one hand and one foot simultaneously, both in a "same-side" pattern (e.g., right hand and right foot) and in an "opposite-side" pattern (e.g., right hand and left foot).

Sara indeed suffered from ataxia, but that didn't explain all of her symptoms. My experience has taught me that a structural defect typically is not, in and of itself, adequate to explain all of a patient's physical or emotional behaviors. In Sara's case, her anxious behavior, coupled with her responses to facilitative and disruptive lenses, led me to the conclusion that her behavior stemmed not just from the damage caused by the injury itself, but also from her emotional reactions to the trauma of that accident.

As neuropsychiatrist Kurt Goldstein notes, such reactions can be cata-strophic—as he puts it, "not only 'inadequate' but also disordered, inconstant, inconsistent and embedded in physical and mental *shock*." In such cases, he notes, "the individual feels himself unfree, buffeted and vac-illating."

Sara's response to yoked prism lenses indicates to me that she can recover to some degree from this trauma, and be restored to a more ordered condition. While she will always have a significant disability due to the damage resulting from her fall, we can help her to perceive her world as a less threatening and more welcoming place. Her prognosis is guarded, but just as she was able to reach out for the balloon after a few moments of wearing the yoked prism lenses, I believe that she eventually can be encouraged to reach out with more confidence to the world around her.

Carlo: A case study revealing why even the wrong lens choice can turn out to be right

So far in this chapter, I've offered case studies in which I was able to select the right yoked prism lenses on the first or second try, based on my clinical observations. That happens most of the time—but even when it doesn't, the results can be enlightening.

Carlo, a two-year-old, is a good example. Nonverbal and highly irritable, Carlo couldn't sit still to watch the video his parents brought. I tried a variety of probes, evaluating his behavior as he sat on his mother's lap, as he ran around, and as I blew bubbles at him. However, he was so tactilely defensive that I was unable to place a pair of lenses on him long enough to evaluate him. The only clue I obtained from my observations was that he displayed a left-sided exotropia.

I told Carlo's parents that given his high stress level, any attempts to force him to pay attention would simply increase his defensiveness, making any findings suspect. Instead, I offered them a loan pair of 2-degree yoked base-up prisms to take home. I told the family not to force Carlo to wear the glasses, but rather to simply keep trying, and to call me for another appointment if they had any success.

In early November, two months after their first visit, Carlo's family called to say that they'd had success in getting him to wear the glasses for an hour or two at a time. They brought him back to the office, and again I had him sit on his mother's lap while watching his favorite video. This time, he was more cooperative. Without the lenses, his head posture tilted to the right, and my immediate thought was, "Base-up was the wrong way to go." I tried yoked base-right lenses instead, and saw an immediate straightening of his head. Yoked base-left was not as successful, and he rejected them, so I returned to the yoked base-right prisms, which he wore without protest.

Next, I asked Carlo to stand on the rocking board. He was so frightened by the movement that I sat him back on his mother's lap for comfort. I put the base-right prisms on him and sat him on the board, and he was able to sit calmly while holding his mother's hand. Eventually he removed his hand and sat independently.

Based on this information and my own clinical experience, I determined that in order to survive, Carlo focused his attention on orienting himself rather than on attending to activity in the space around him. This type of behavior leads to great anxiety, both in individuals considered "normal" and in those with developmental disabilities. Without intervention, as such individuals grow into adulthood, these anxieties persist and usually increase. In such individuals, the neuromotor system compresses "self" and space to such a degree that it stops all eye movement.

When the wrong lenses were applied to Carlo, they forced him to immediately reorganize his neural system, leading to movement changes and improved visual capture (the ability to visually "grab on to" information). These changes enabled him to take the first steps out of his shell. If left on too long, however, the wrong lenses would have caused negative changes in the visual system. Once I determined that Carlo performed best with base-right prisms, I sent him home with a prescription for these lenses, which will foster the long-term changes that will lead to permanent improvements in his visual behavior.

The key point of Carlo's story is that "wrong" responses to lenses should not be judged as failures. Under analysis, these responses may give us insight into an individual's adaptive reactions.

Israel Greenwald, O.D., who practices in Staten Island, is an expert in the treatment of strabismus. As part of his treatment he uses large-magnitude disruptive prisms as an "overcorrection" technique to increase motor neuron activity, often leading to the sudden and deliberate repositioning of a strabismic eye. This same reasoning helps to explain why the use of disruptive yoked prisms can cause an immediate, positive response, by forcing the patient's brain to immediately change ingrained patterns of visual behavior. It also explains why one task does not make a diagnosis. Instead, you must observe the reactions of a patient for a period of time (sometimes, as in Carlo's case, an extended period), under the demands of different tasks.

Explaining prism lenses to patients and their families

Selecting prism lenses takes time, patience, and careful observation. Once you have accomplished this task, it is equally important to educate patients or their caretakers about the rationale for using these lenses. Most people who consult you for vision therapy will know little or nothing about what yoked prism lenses are, and how they affect vision. Thus, you'll want to allow ample time to explain why you are prescribing the lenses, and what you expect them to do (see a sample explanation below).

Be sure to allow plenty of time for patients or caretakers to ask questions, and invite them to call if they have additional questions or concerns before their next visit. The relationship between therapist and patient is often a long-term one, and educating and supporting your patients or their families will help to start that relationship on the right foot.

What to tell your patients about yoked prism lenses

My discussions with patients or caretakers vary, depending on each individual's interest and level of knowledge, but I typically offer an explanation similar to this:

You have just received a very carefully prescribed pair of glasses. They probably look like any other pair you've seen and may have worn. Actually, they're quite different, and even have a different purpose.

Almost all glasses have what is called "compensating lenses," because that's exactly what they do—compensate for some inadequacy in the way an eye performs.

If something gets blurry when it comes up close, or is far away, compensating lenses sharpen up the image. Or they can help eyes adapt to the way light comes in. They can even help to uncross crossed eyes.

In essence, they clear up sight.

These glasses of yours do that, of course. But they also do something else. They have what are called "therapeutic lenses." Their purpose is not just to compensate for a problem, but also to create change.

Right now your eyes are not working as a team, or at least not together as a team. And they aren't working effectively as "players" in your total mind/body complex.

Imagine what that means to how you function throughout the day. One eye may be sending one kind of information to the brain, while the other is sending something different. Or it may be that the brain is overwhelmed by the fears and "body schema" problems that vision problems can cause.

When your brain can't trust your eyes, it has to make some decisions. Should it act on the information from your eyes, or reject that information and instead use the input from other body senses? Think of an orchestra, in which all of the musicians are playing separately. You'd hear noise, not music.

Right now, your brain is working as hard to sort out the information it's getting as it is to do the task you're asking of it, whether that task is reading, playing sports, painting, sewing, or watching television. That sorting out of information takes energy—energy you could be using to do reading, or playing, or painting, or sewing, or watching. If that energy were available to you, you could get more done, in less time, with less strain.

Your new glasses will train your eyes to work together. That's why they're called "therapeutic," and why you'll only be wearing them for a prescribed amount of time.

While you wear these glasses, they will literally reorganize your vision. As a result, your brain won't have to do that difficult sorting job anymore. Eventually, your eyes will become so accustomed to working together they won't need outside help anymore. When the eyes lead the mind, your performance is enhanced. When the mind leads the eyes—as yours does right now—it interferes.

How long it will take for you to see benefits will depend on you, your specific problem, and how long it has been a problem. In some cases this schedule is predictable, and in other cases, only time will tell. Visual training, in many cases, will speed the process. When lenses alone are prescribed, we'll see you again in two months for a progress examination to see how much improvement there has been. At that point, we'll be able to give you a better idea.

You may have some things to tell us, too. You're likely to find, as most people do, that many things are becoming easier for you to do, even in that short a time. That's because every day your brain will get more used to focusing on the tasks you want it to do, instead of spending excess energy struggling to sort out information.

Notes

1   Information on interpreting these results is included in "Vertical yoked prisms: Testing and use of Kaplan System for prescribing vertical yoked prisms," in M. Kaplan and F. Flach (2000), "Infant and Toddler Strabismus and Amblyopia: Behavioral Aspects of Vision Care." *Optometric Extension Program 41*, 2.

2   Following a typical pattern, Tony's listening skills improved before his speech appeared. These language skills do not develop in parallel because the speech–auditory complex is divided, with the auditory system handling receptive language and the speech system handling the complex skills required for expression. (The visual system is the only single modality that has both receptive and expressive ability.) When our patients become better at using their eye movements efficiently, it takes far less effort for them to attend to and orchestrate sensory input. This leaves the cortex with more time to analyze language, resulting first in better passive receptive skills and later in the development of the cognitive, motor, and coordination skills needed for speech.

Part III

Planning a Visual Management Program

CHAPTER 5

The Therapy Process:
A Philosophical Overview

Early physicians accurately described the physiology of the eye well before the time of Galen. However, the *function* of the eye was poorly understood until Johannes Kepler published a paper in 1604 showing that the eye works by focusing an image on the retina—or, in more modern terms, that it works like a camera.

The comparison of the eye to a camera is relevant for another reason: a picture taken by a camera has no meaning except as it is *interpreted* by an individual, based on that person's perception, intelligence, and past experiences. Similarly, vision is not simply the process of "taking a picture" with the eye. To truly *see* requires a sophisticated construction of visual intelligence whose intricacies are still being unfolded by neuropsychologists and physiologists.

We construct the parts of our universe into a coherent whole in many ways, using color, motion, shapes, texture, and prior experience. Individuals with autism spectrum disorders, other developmental problems, or mental illnesses—and, to a lesser degree, children with learning disabilities—have visual impairments that interfere with this process, thus limiting their visual intelligence. The problem is not that their eyes cannot "take a picture"; rather, the problem is that they cannot perceive this picture correctly, and thus cannot act on it logically.

A good illustration of this involves a patient of mine named Ned, whose diagnosis could be considered as "functional" dorsal simultanagnosia. Individuals with dorsal simultanagnosia, which usually stems from a head injury, are unable to recognize two or more objects or parts of objects at the same time. They can see motions and edges with normal acuity, and can assemble them visually into a whole, but can see only one object or part of an object at a time.

Ned, a 26-year-old graduate student, exhibited a similar problem, but his symptoms were related to mental illness rather than a head injury. He was quite brilliant, but his education was interrupted by many hospital stays for emotional disturbance. While in therapy, he became more stable, and could attend school successfully.

About three months into Ned's therapy, I was interviewed for a newspaper article and the reporter asked if she could interview some of my patients. Ned happened to be in a session at that time and agreed to talk with her. Later, she told me that she'd asked him, "How has vision management helped you?" He replied, "Before Dr. Kaplan's therapy, if I was out in a street I would look at a car and I could see only a door handle, a headlight, a tire—and I would have to construct in my mind that it was a car. Now when I look, I see the car."

There was nothing wrong with Ned's eyes prior to therapy, but there was a great deal wrong with his nervous system's interpretation of what his eyes saw. As a result, the simplest visual activities required enormous mental effort, sapping his energy and making academic and personal achievements a struggle.

Similarly, my patients often have "perfect" sight for vision, but their brains cannot make sense of what their eyes are telling them. This impairment has a devastating effect, because once we are born, our future development depends to a large degree on what we see, hear, touch, and do—and, even more importantly, on how accurately our brains are able to integrate and interpret this information. When this process of perception breaks down, so does our ability to form an accurate picture of our space world, to interact with that world successfully, to master each stage of development, and to form the memories that will allow us to survive and thrive in the future. The result, as in Ned's case, is a constant struggle to survive, leaving little or no time and energy for growth and learning.

Fortunately for our patients, it is possible to retrain the brain to quickly and easily understand the information that the eyes are sending—to "see the car," as Ned would put it—rather than fighting to make sense of incomprehensible images. It is possible, too, to jump-start developmental processes that have been stalled by visual impairments, as dysfunctional adaptations are unlearned and new and more functional perceptual patterns are established.

Prism lenses begin this process, by instantly altering perception and awakening dormant neural processes. To truly improve our patients' visual performance, however, we must provide long-term therapy that will enable them to transform the temporary changes brought about by prism lenses into permanent neural alteration. Such transformations lead not just to better vision, but also to better physical, emotional, and cognitive ability. This concept—that improvement in visual intelligence leads to greater well-being in every facet of behavior and performance—has been the basis for developmental vision therapy since its inception.

A brief history of vision therapy

As I noted in Chapter 2, A.M. Skeffington is rightly credited as the "father of behavioral optometry." However, I was startled to learn recently that the connection between dysfunctional vision and dysfunctional behavior, a concept I'd always believed to be fairly new—and one that is a cornerstone of modern developmental optometry—was originally made more than a century and a half ago by Edouard Seguin.

Seguin, a famous physician in his time, devoted much of his life to treating developmentally disabled patients—or, in the unfortunate idiom of the time, "idiots." He had considerable success, considering the lack of knowledge about mental disorders at the time, in educating children formerly thought to be beyond help.

While many of Seguin's ideas now seem archaic, he was far ahead of his time in identifying the disturbed visual processes of his developmentally disabled patients. In his most famous work, *Idiocy: and its Treatment by the Physiological Method,* he recognized the role of vision in behavior, and tentatively grasped the concept of visual deficits as adaptations to neurological deficits (that is, "software" rather than "hardware" problems), when he wrote of his patients:

> The Sight may be as badly and more ostentatiously impaired than the hearing. Be it fixed in one canthus, be it wandering and unfixable, be it glossy, laughing, like a picture moving behind a motionless varnish, be it dull and immured to images, its meanings are not doubtful; it means idiocy. Our expressions here would be very incorrect if they

conveyed the idea that these defects of vision prevent the child from seeing. The images being printed on their passing into the ocular chamber, as the river-side scenery is on the passing current, the child, when he pays an accidental attention, gets a notion of some of them, but the transitory perception produced thereby can hardly serve him for educational purposes. The principal characters of this infirmity are, the repugnance of the child to look and the incapacity of his will to control the organs of vision; he sees by chance, but never looks. These defects of the sight, when grave, are always connected with automatic motions, and both oppose serious obstacles to progress; one by the ease with which the child can use his negative will to prevent the training of his eyes, the other by depriving him of all knowledge to be acquired farther than the touch can reach.[1]

In Seguin's early observations, we see the roots of our current knowledge that visual problems often stem not from structural defects, but from a patient "shutting down" visual processes in order to cope with an overwhelming world.

Based on Seguin's observations of visual and other sensory deficits in his patients, he incorporated rudimentary sensory therapy into their regimens—perhaps the first instance of sensory integration therapy being practiced in the United States. Although his approaches probably were of only limited value to his patients, because of the dearth of knowledge about neurological development available at the time, Seguin deserves great credit for identifying the role of impaired sensory processes in behavioral disturbance.

Seguin was also the first clinician to recognize the importance of incorporating movement into therapy. In the 1800s, Seguin noted that because people with developmental disabilities frequently do not respond to their exterior senses, the clinician must begin by educating their internal senses on a physiological level in order to restore harmony. He wrote, "Let it be one of our first duties to correct the automatic motions, and supply the deficiencies of the muscular apparatus; otherwise how could we expect to ripen a crop of intellectual faculties on a field obstructed by disordered functions?"

Unfortunately, Seguin's foresighted ideas about the incorporation of visual, sensory, and movement therapies into the treatment of patients with developmental delays or mental illnesses received little attention from other practitioners for many decades. However, the use of vision therapy for the general population continued to gain in popularity, as both doctors and patients discovered its benefits. In 1865, about the time that Seguin was writing about his work, Louis Javal—credited with being the first practitioner of orthoptics—introduced therapy based on eye exercises. Javal is also notable as the first doctor to use the stereoscope to treat strabismus.

Skeffington, of course, deserves particular recognition as an early leader in the field of visual management, for introducing the use of lenses as a learning tool, and for recognizing the fact that visual ability can be improved through training (see Chapter 2). As I've noted, Skeffington is considered the father of modern vision therapy, and his seminal "four circles" model (Figure 2.1) established the concept of vision as a dynamic, integrative process. Another important step occurred many decades later, when Arneson identified the importance of peripheral (ambient) stimulation in visual training.

It was in the 1950s and 1960s, however, that much of the progress in modern behavioral vision therapy occurred, a great deal of it at the Gesell Institute. It was at this facility, for example, that Gerald Getman—who laid the groundwork for much of modern-day visual training—developed a structured program of vision therapy based on the concept that visual perception is not just a product of the eyes and brain, but a product of the entire bodily experience. Getman recognized that the development of gross motor skills is a prerequisite for the development of perceptual skills, and his training focused on guiding patients through six stages of motor and perceptual development. These are:

1. *General movement patterns:* Overall generalized movement, and the improvement of hand–eye coordination. This is the first step in fostering perceptual skills.

2. *Special movement patterns:* Refinement and extension of movements, further preparing an individual for perceptual tasks.

3. *Eye movement patterns:* The use of vision to replace general or special movements, freeing the hands for more productive uses.

4. *Communications or visual language patterns:* The use of speech to replace the need for action.

5. *Visualization pattern:* "Visual memory," or the recall of previously learned information, the analysis of things already known, and the inspection of new information.

6. *Visual perceptual organization:* The ability to interchangeably use speech, vision, and movement to interpret the environment.

Getman's work formed the basis for much of modern visual training. A key aspect of his philosophy was that perceptual and motor skills cannot be viewed as two separate activities because each provides continual feedback to the other, allowing an organism to coordinate motor movements and spatial apprehension. Getman's ideas underlie today's awareness that vision is not a static and isolated process, but rather an active and holistic process that affects, and is affected by, every system of the body.

The method of vision therapy that I practice builds heavily on the work of Getman and his colleagues, but with refinements based both on my clinical experience and on scientific findings since their time. For instance, Getman asserted that the development of efficient perceptual and motor feedback loops depended primarily upon the learning of gross motor skills. Clinically, however, this is only a half truth. In reality, perception and motor skills are mutually dependent. Delays in gross motor skills force the individual to pay greater attention to orientation, reducing the energy available to attend spatial cues. This reduces the individual's ability to explore and learn from the environment, which in turn affects future visual competence.

Another difference between my conceptual approach to vision therapy and Getman's concerns his insistence that if a stage of development is not attained, failure will be experienced at higher stages. This concept has merit but it is a bit of an exaggeration because other factors often come into play, including innate intelligence, and emotional resilience. I often see "overcompensated" high achievers who have mastered higher-level skills while missing basic building blocks, although they do so at a great cost of effort and energy.

In Getman's view, disorders in gross motor skills need to be corrected before training in visual perception is undertaken. The underlying idea is that development is sequential and orderly. In reality, however, development is never even, and the proper order of therapy is more logically dictated by the strengths, motivation, and perceptual style of each patient, as well as the embeddedness of the visual processing system.

This is particularly true when dealing with patients on the autistic spectrum, who exhibit markedly uneven developmental patterns. One reason for this, according to new research,[2] is that individual regions in the autistic brain function normally or even in a superior manner, but these regions fail to "network" as well as they do in the brains of non-disabled people. This results, quite often, in remarkable performance in skills that require an isolated brain area—for instance, perfect pitch or an amazing ability in art—combined with severe deficits in other areas, such as language or postural control, which require synchronicity. It also results in highly idiosyncratic patterns of development. Rather than trying to force individuals with autism to conform to a developmental chart, it is far more effective for the clinician to tailor therapy to their individual strengths and weaknesses.

Key principles of vision therapy

I am often asked, "What activities would you recommend for a child with such-and-such a problem?" As with selecting prism lenses, there is no single correct answer to this question. The tools used in my office (pegboards, balls, puzzles, musical instruments, etc.) are for the most part the same as you'll find in the office of any vision therapist. Similarly, while I've devised many original activities to help patients, most of my training procedures are based on well-established techniques used for years by developmental optometrists. The skill lies less in the tools and exercises themselves than in evaluating each patient correctly, and then selecting appropriate activities based on three criteria:

- What is the demand of the task?
- Does the task have meaning to this particular patient?
- Can this task lead to a higher level of proficiency?

Selecting the appropriate tasks for each patient, and presenting them in the correct order, is an art that requires clinical judgment and experience, as well as an understanding of the goals and structure of an effective therapy program. The following four guiding principles, discussed at length below, will aid in planning therapy that will help each patient to achieve his or her maximum potential:

1. Vision therapy is more than just "fixing eyes," and the therapist cannot address vision in isolation.

2. Movement is central to any therapy plan.

3. Vision therapy must be consistent with a patient's abilities and perceptual style.

4. Therapy moves through logical stages.

Vision therapy is more than just "fixing eyes"

For patients to achieve a true feeling of normalcy, vision therapy needs to be not just intrasensory (focusing on vision alone) but intersensory (involving the integration of all senses). The systematic training of the individual as a whole is more useful and faster than correction of a single action.

In effect, our job is not just to fix our patients' vision but, more holistically, to fix their entire view of themselves and their world. As Michael Gazzaniga noted in *The Social Brain*,[3] one of the main jobs of consciousness is to keep our lives tied together into a coherent story—in other words, a self-concept. It does this by generating explanations of behavior on the basis of our self-image, memories of the past, expectations of the future, our current social situation, and our physical environment. In the case of our patients, all of these explanations are flawed, and must be "re-written" to reflect a new perceptual reality.

This rewriting is a global process, and if we try to change a patient's performance by viewing any one system in isolation, we will be constructing incomplete mind images and the patient will substitute one organization of constraints for another. Therefore, when we implement visual management procedures, our goal is to incorporate the total neuromotor complex, rather than vision in isolation.

Movement is central to any therapy plan

Movement is an integral part of any visual management program, because human beings are "spatial action units" and movement is the basis of awareness. Difficulties in movement undermine and distort performance, and lead to behaviors that interfere with natural development. When we break dysfunctional habits of movement, and force patients to learn new and more efficient patterns, we see a resulting improvement in eye movement and visual skills. As Moshe Feldenkrais, developer of the highly regarded Feldenkrais Method of Somatic Education, states,

> A fundamental change in the motor basis within any single integration pattern will break up the cohesion of the whole and thereby leave thought and feeling without anchorage in the patterns of their established routines. In this condition it is much easier to effect changes in thinking and feeling, for the muscular part through which thinking and feeling reach our awareness has changed and no longer expresses the patterns previously familiar to us. Habit has lost its chief support, that of the muscles, and has become more amenable to change.[4]

To be effective, vision therapy must break old patterns, and stimulate a patient to move, feel, and think. One procedure that accomplishes this goal is Disruptive Lazy Eight (described in Chapter 7), a procedure using spatial rearrangement to consciously stimulate awareness of what the patient sees and feels. Another good example is a procedure I use to aid patients in mastering directionality (the ability to discriminate right from left). This skill is critical, because in order for individuals to know where objects are in relation to "self," they must first know where they themselves are. To address postural deficits and related issues, we must allow our patients to establish what Roelofs, the researcher and vision expert, described as "that centre, fixed with reference to the body, from which absolute directions are judged, such as straight ahead, to the left, to the right, upward or downward."[5]

Normally, as noted by Piaget, children learn to discriminate right from left on their own bodies by the time they are six, although they are unable to determine right and left on other people before the age of eight. In addressing the directional difficulties of verbal children, I have great success moving these children through egocentricity to lateral movement awareness in feeling and seeing—and then on to the integration of moving, seeing, and thinking—using the Tai Chi-type movement described below.

Tai Chi—Tai Chi standing

Materials

Chalkboard

Chalk and erasers

Set-up

On the chalkboard, draw one row of arrows: up, down, right, and left. Direct the patient to stand in front of and facing the chalkboard, approximately 5 feet away.

Procedure

The patient performs a series of movements coordinated with breathing, according to the directions depicted by the arrows. The first arrow points up. The patient should raise both arms up over his or her head while blowing out a long, even, relaxed breath. The patient should fully extend both arms over the head. As the patient returns both arms to his or her sides, he or she should pull in a deep breath.

The next arrow points down. The patient should blow out a smooth, even breath while bringing both arms down in a relaxed and flowing motion. The patient should then pull in a deep breath while bringing the arms back to the starting point.

The third arrow points to the right. The patient should bring his or her right arm to the right until it is fully extended, while at the same time blowing out in a smooth and even manner. As the patient brings the right arm back to the starting point, he or she should pull the breath back in.

The last arrow points to the left. The patient should bring his or her left arm to the left until it is fully extended, while at the same time blowing out in a smooth and even manner. As the patient brings the left arm back to the starting point, he or she should pull the breath back in.

The interaction of visual, kinesthetic and breathing modalities in this procedure is associated with a reactivation of the postural reflexes, leading to an improved sense of directionality, which in turn enhances a wide range of skills ranging from reading to social interaction. The procedure can also be performed, with modifications, by nonverbal patients, who respond equally well.

Another good example of integrating motion into vision therapy is an eye tracking exercise I frequently use in my office to treat strabismus. This activity is performed in a supine position, using a Marsden ball that swings in a pendulum-like motion up and down the length of the patient's body. The patient is asked to actively feel his or her eyes as they move while watching the ball, and to point to the ball as it moves. (I ask whether this activity is easier with or without the patient pointing, and pick the easier route.) The patient is then asked to close his or her eyes and continue tracking by imagining where the ball is as it swings, while again actively feeling the movement of the eyes. Periodically, the patient opens his or her eyes to check the accuracy of his or her perception. This exercise is repeated with the ball swinging side to side across the body, and then with the patient sitting and finally standing. The perception of movement awareness is accomplished through the interaction of the visual, kinesthetic and tactile modalities, while slowly bringing into action the postural reflex. When I ask patients to engage in these and similar activities, I am creating movement awareness through perceptual rearrangement. The result is a change in perceptual-motor coordination leading to more effective integration between perceptual modalities. This frequently results in rapid and positive changes.

Some readers may question why so much emphasis is placed in this book on the lower-level nervous system function of movement, when the vision therapist is addressing higher-level processes of vision and hearing and cognition. The reason is quite simple. The nervous system is hierarchical, and in order for the higher levels of the central nervous system to solve a problem quickly, the organism's lower-level functions must be reflexive.

In simple terms, the nervous system is organized much like an army. To be efficient, this army must be able to delegate the routine tasks of movement to the privates and sergeants and corporals, freeing the officers to make more complex decisions. When lower-level processes fail,

Some time ago I conducted an initial training session with Sharon, a nine-year-old girl who suffered from learning and movement problems that interfered with her academic and social life. Watching Sharon's therapy, her father interrupted to ask, "How will I know if the lenses and therapy are working?"

Previously, I had observed Sharon's behavior as she read a book out loud. I said to her father, "Your daughter rocks forward and backward in a continual, rhythmic motion when she reads. How long has she exhibited this rocking behavior?" He replied that she'd rocked when reading ever since preschool, adding that the family had tried different interventions with no success. I asked him, "If Sharon's rocking stopped, would that be a fair indicator that vision training is working?" He answered, "Of course."

The therapist began working with Sharon again, using a simple tracking sequence involving eye and hand movement integrated with breathing. At the end of the sequence, I asked Sharon to read again. This time she read faster and more loudly than before, and she did not rock at all. Even I was surprised at how quickly her rocking stopped, as I had anticipated that this would take a month or so of therapy. Watching Sharon read, her father said, "I am a believer."

the principle of "least interaction" is violated, and the colonels and generals—vision, hearing, and other higher-level processes—must step in, leaving less time and energy for their proper functions. When we remediate movement problems, we free the higher levels of the nervous system to perform their own jobs more quickly and efficiently. As a result, a patient who moves more naturally will also be able to see, hear, and think better.

One key in addressing movement problems is the concept of *synergy*. Mathematician and biologist I.M. Gelfand described synergies as "classes of movements that have similar kinematic characteristics, coinciding active muscle groups, and conducting types of afferentation."[6] In simpler terms, synergies involve groups of muscles acting in a unified manner in response to environmental demands, making them far more efficient than if they were to act alone. Nicholas O'Dwyer, of the School of Exercise and Sport Science at the University of Sydney, offers a good example of synergy:

Arutyanyan *et al.* found that in unskilled [shooters], movement at one joint was not compensated by a change at the other joint, thus throwing the gun off target. The two joints were relatively independent of each other. But in a skilled marksperson, the two joints were constrained to act as a unit such that any horizontal oscillation in the wrist was matched by an equal and opposite horizontal oscillation of the shoulder. In the skilled person it appears that the joints related among themselves according to some equation of constraint, whereas in the unskilled person, the joints appeared to vary in a relatively independent fashion, meaning that no equation of constraint applied. The skilled person had learned to constrain the joints to operate as a single functional unit or coordinative structure. Learning any skill probably entails a similar discovery of relevant constraints over the joints and muscles used in the skill.[7]

A lack of synergy is responsible for many symptoms associated with walking, running, writing, or sports activities. A good illustration is the midline problems that are almost universal in people with autism.[8] When evaluating an autistic child, ask the child to lie on his or her back, arms at the side, legs together, and then to move the limbs you touch in a sweeping "angels in the snow" pattern. Some patients will not be able to move at all. Others will move only one limb at a time. Still others will be able to move an arm and leg on the same side of the body. None, in my experience, can move heterogeneously (right arm/left leg or left arm/right leg). This is evidence of a lack of synergistic classes of movement.

In discussing synergies, Gelfand compared them to a "dictionary of movement." Expanding on this analogy, we can say that the efforts of individual muscles are letters of the language of movements, and synergies combine these letters into words, which carry far more meaning than individual jumbles of letters. Children with autism spectrum disorders or other developmental disabilities have a limited "dictionary" of synergies. As a result, they do not have time to visually interpret the abundance of cues in their surroundings, and must resort to slower senses of touch, taste, and smell in order to interact with the complexities of their environment.

Synergy, like other developmental skills, is learned by experience, and therefore can be changed by experience. Prism lenses set the playing field for visual improvement by altering perception, but it is visual training that creates synergies. Over time, these synergies consolidate, become automatic, and can be consistently executed in an appropriate time frame. Like coaches who advise players that "If you have to think, you've already lost," visual management experts know that it is the preparation of movement synergies, and the resulting automaticity, that allow a patient to succeed.

Some of the cases I describe in this book involve patients with such simplicity of synergistic actions that they can move only one muscle group at a time. In these cases, the "hammer" of disruptive lenses is much more effective than the "feather" of facilitative lenses. These patients possess such restricted movement and visual attention that change requires a perceived threat to their very survival. In these cases, vision therapy using both yoked prism and vision therapy creates a "readiness for movement," preparing patients for kinesthetic and visual stimulation in a directive or disruptive manner. Initially, disruptive lenses may create fear, distrust, and avoidance. However, with training, patients begin to feel their self-induced constraints falling away. Their awareness of expanding spatial cues stimulates new synergies, and the "aha" of realization often leads to a tremendous sense of euphoria.

One of the most important synergies the therapist must address is that of the hands and the eyes. My own observations, as well as those of Edouard Seguin in the 1800s, reveal that individuals with developmental disabilities have problems in prehension, or the use of the hands (seizing, grasping). It is common in the delayed and autistic population to see individuals hold their hands in fists, sometimes so tight that their fingers appear gnarled.

This constraint in the use of the hands has repercussions on the development of visual skills as well. From birth, a child learns to reach, grasp, and release—skills paralleled by development of the visual system, which forms neural patterns that visually reach for an object, explore it, and release it visually and saccadically move on. Later, as the child grips a pencil for writing, or catches and throws a ball, the hands lead the eyes to track and change from one target to another. As the child moves from general to specific movements, there is greater complexity in moving the hand than in moving the rest of the body, which is why it takes time to learn advanced grasp-and-release skills such as using a fork, holding a pencil, or buttoning a shirt.

Children with developmental delays often learn to reach and grasp, but never progress to the ability to release. While most new parents are proud when their baby strongly grasps a finger and won't let go, releasing is a more advanced stage and one that is crucial both for exploration and for development of the visual system. Thus, one of my first goals in working with a child with poor release skills is to use bodily movement to relax the hand, which allows the hand to lead the eye and later allows the eye to lead the hand.

Cheri, a four-year-old with autism, refused to even step on the rocking board in my office. Based on my evaluation, which showed that Cheri had a tunneled perceptual style, I prescribed 3-diopter base-down yoked prisms.

After starting Cheri on a gentle rolling exercise to stimulate her vestibular system, I next prescribed a five-minute rocking procedure to be done twice a day. In this procedure, Cheri's mother sat on the floor facing a mirror, with Cheri sitting between her mother's legs and facing forward. Cheri held a dowel horizontally in both hands, with her mother's hands placed over hers for guidance. Cheri's mother rocked from side to side, gently moving Cheri as well. Initially, Cheri kept her fingers tightly fisted and paid no visual attention to herself in the mirror. (Children with a "tunneled" perceptual style, like Cheri, need to monitor themselves in the mirror in order to be anchored.) Over time, however, Cheri's hands began to relax, and simultaneously she began to pay more attention to herself in the mirror. By the end of the week, she was secure enough to rock without her mother or the stick, while viewing herself in the mirror.

The second week, I asked Cheri's mother to sit behind her daughter as Cheri sat on a rocking board facing a mirror. As in the previous exercise, Cheri held the dowel and her mother, also holding the dowel, guided her to rock gently. Cheri responded more quickly this time, relaxing her hands and paying attention to her reflection, and by the end of the week she could sit and rock independently while watching her reflection. The third week we repeated this exercise with Cheri standing on the rocking board, again with quick success.

I saw similar progress with Dylan, a teenager with multiple disabilities who displayed a total lack of balance on the rocking board. Like Cheri, Dylan tended to hold his hands tightly clenched. I had him stand on the rocking board holding the dowel, while his mother stood in front of him with her hands guiding the dowel as he rocked. After a few minutes of guidance, Dylan was able to continue rocking as his mother let go. A minute or two later, he began attending to the video, and his hands began to relax. This was the first small but important step in what proved to be a highly successful therapy program, with Dylan eventually making remarkable strides in visual performance and, as a result, in physical and academic skills.

There is no limit to the tools we can use to stimulate hand movement and hand–eye coordination in our patients. Gerald Getman, in *Developing Your Child's Intelligence,*[9] recommends giving children old coffee pots and other safe gadgets with multiple parts, and letting them explore with their eyes and hands how to manipulate these items, take them apart, and put them back together. In my office, I use a wide variety of puzzles, pegboards, string beads, and musical instruments. The choice of tool is less important than the goal of moving the patient from immobility to mobility, which will heighten visual perception.

Another critical synergy involves movement and breathing. For many of my patients, dysfunctional breathing has such an impact on visual processes that little progress can be made in therapy until natural, efficient breathing is restored. This topic is so important that I have devoted an entire chapter to it later in this book (see Chapter 9).

Vision therapy must be consistent with a patient's abilities and perceptual style

In planning a therapy approach, goals and procedures must be based on a realistic evaluation of each patient's strengths and weaknesses. An effective program of vision therapy is based not just on the patient's response to yoked prism lenses, but also on the patient's age, maturity, attitude, attention span, competence in expressive and receptive language, and perceptual style. (For instance, I have discovered in my own practice that patients with global perceptual styles are more comfortable when they self-initiate. Patients with focal perceptual styles, conversely, typically prefer to be directed.)

The design of a therapy program should also be based on whether the patient's perceptual style involves "flight" or "fight." Our patients are rarely conscious of the way they see, hear, or touch, but they are very aware of their fears and anxieties, which in many cases dominate their performance and behavior. Some patients choose the "flight" response: for instance, the hysterical amblyopic patient who loses visual acuity for emotional reasons, the child who shuts his eyes when objects are thrown at him, or the child who covers her ears at a certain point when watching a video. Others choose the "fight" response, succeeding at each task but only through determination and an extreme expenditure of energy: for instance, the learning-disabled child who studies an extra three hours each night just to keep up, or the child with Asperger Syndrome who struggles determinedly to fit in socially. Identifying a patient's perceptual style is a key part of developing a therapy program that will allow your patient to achieve maximal performance without becoming overwhelmed, and to sustain these gains when training is finished.

It is also important to determine whether a patient's most severe problems involve orientation (sense of self) or organization (sense of surrounding space). "Self" is what one feels, while space is what one sees. Monitoring "self" requires attention to proprioceptive cues, while monitoring space requires attention to visual cues. Orientation and organization should interact and maintain a balance; when this does not happen, the patient develops constraints in order to adapt. The best approach is to address the most impaired of the two processes at the outset of therapy, bringing them back into balance.

Therapy moves through logical stages

Vision therapy using yoked prism lenses is based on stimulating consciousness, either in a directive or disruptive manner, in order to allow patients to reach a higher level of visual performance. This process moves through three logical stages, each building on the previous one. These stages are *awareness*, *attention*, and *automacity*.

Awareness is, in effect, a neural "awakening." Movie buffs may recall the Robert De Niro film *Awakenings* in which De Niro played a comatose patient brought back to consciousness by a chemical treatment. The film re-created the real-life professional experience of neurologist Oliver Sacks, who stimulated a temporary neural awakening in patients who had been comatose (some for decades) as a result of encephalitis, when he administered the drug L-dopa to them.

In the case of Sacks' patients, this awakening lasted only briefly before they slipped back into irreversible comas. The awareness we create in vision therapy, however, is real and lasting, because we are actually permanently altering neural function. This results in our patients becoming aware of the input from all of their senses, and aware of their own motor responses to this stimulation. It allows them to actively perceive, remember, and respond to events in their environment.

The next step in patients' progress is an improvement in *attention*. At this stage, patients become more capable of allocating and focusing energy. This requires a higher level of performance than awareness, because the act of paying attention creates neural stress and requires accurate visual perception.

The third step in training is *automacity*, in which patients become able to perform tasks while paying little active attention. When individuals are in harmony with their world, their actions become reflexive. An obvious example is the act of driving, which is enormously stressful for a novice, but can be done almost on "autopilot" by an experienced driver. At this level, awareness actually impedes performance, because it interferes with unconscious synergies of movement.

It is crucial for training to be long term, so that patients can move from awareness to attention to automacity. This is necessary in order for them to achieve the highest possible level of performance.

On a more concrete level, the individual activities that make up a program of vision therapy must also be based on a logical hierarchy. In designing a program of therapy for individuals with autism or other disabilities, the clinician should structure procedures to proceed logically through these three stages:

- guidance, in which the therapist demonstrates the task

- imitation, in which the therapist demonstrates the task and then asks the patient to imitate the action, offering assistance as needed

- initiation, the highest level of performance, in which the patient can perform the task independently with no prompting.

A good example of breaking a task into these three stages is a time-honored procedure I call "Pie Tin Rotation." This activity, which improves hand—eye coordination by requiring simultaneous movement of wrists, hands, and eyes, is highly motivating for children with autism spectrum disorders because it asks them to track a continuous movement of a ball or toy car. This is a focal task, much like watching spinning wheels or running water, which children with autism find appealing.

The therapist introduces this task by sitting across from the child, holding a pie tin and placing a 2½-inch ball or toy car in it. The therapist then moves the pie tin very slowly, so the ball or toy rolls slowly around the perimeter of the tin's bottom. In nearly every case, the child will become interested in the movement, and reach out to grab the car or ball. At this point, the therapist allows the child to inspect the object, and then places it back in the tin. This time, the therapist places the child's hands on the edge of the tin, uses his or her own hands to guide the child in moving the tin to make the ball or car roll around the edge, and then encourages the child to imitate the action. Eventually, as the therapist fades his or her prompting, the child will begin to make the ball spin independently. (This task can be altered to involve rolling two balls or cars around the inner edge of the tin, while keeping the two objects separated. This requires slow, controlled movements, and a higher level of attention. To add more difficulty, the activity can be done standing.) By structuring a task in this manner, we allow a patient to move from dependence to independence, without risk of failure.

Depending on a patient's developmental level, it may not be necessary to provide guidance or hands-on assistance. Verbal, higher-functioning patients may need little or no help before performing even a challenging task independently. Lower-functioning patients, however, will nearly always need to work through all three steps of guidance, imitation, and initiation. The key for any patient is to start at a level that will guarantee interest and success, and avoid frustration.

One additional logical progression in therapy is to begin with patients' strengths and progress toward their weaknesses. Again, this reduces the chances of failure, and encourages and motivates patients. A "clinical pearl" in this regard: patients who ground themselves by using proprioceptive cues do best when they can self-observe using a mirror, while patients who rely on spatial cues attend best while watching television or other external objects. When working with patients who prefer proprioceptive cues, I begin by having them perform dowel stick procedures, Simon Says, and balance board activities while facing a mirror. When working with patients who prefer spatial cues, I begin with television-watching or activities in which they imitate the therapist.

Patients often have problems in both orientation and spatial organization, but typically they will show greater impairment in one area than the other. As I noted earlier, therapy should be planned to focus initially on either orientation or organization, depending on which is causing the greatest difficulty for the patient.

In keeping with this approach, the remainder of this part of the book is divided into one chapter dealing with orientation, and a second dealing with spatial organization. These are followed by a chapter on the very important topic of breathing. Before discussing these aspects of therapy, however, I will devote some attention to one of the most common problems that we see in optometry, and one of the most controversial: strabismus.

Notes

1   Seguin, E. (1866) *Idiocy: and its Treatment by the Physiological Method*. New York: William Wood and Co.

2   Just, M.A., Cherkasskym V.L., Keller, T.A. and Minshew, N.J. (2004) "Cortical activation and synchronization during sentence comprehension in high-functioning autism: Evidence of underconnectivity." *Brain 127*, 8, 1811–1821.

3   Gazzaniga, M. (1985) *The Social Brain: Discovering the Networks of the Mind*. New York: Basic Books.

4   Feldenkrais, M. (1980) *Awareness Through Movement: Health Exercises for Personal Growth*. London: Penguin Books.

5   Roelofs, C.O. (1959) "Considerations on the visual egocentre." *Acta Psychology 16*, 226–234.

6   Gelfand, I.M. (1971) "Some problems in the analysis of movements." In *Models of the Structural–Functional Organization of Certain Biological Systems*. Edited by I.M. Gelfand with V.S. Gurfinkel, S.V. Fomin and M.L. Tsetlin. Cambridge MA: MIT Press.

7   O'Dwyer, N. "Coordination, degrees of freedom and synergies." Lecture available from www2.fhs.usyd.edu.

8   There is a correlation between midline problems in the body and coordination of the eyes. All strabismics have a midline problem, as do individuals with vergence dysfunction.

9   Getman, G.N. (1984) *How to Develop Your Child's Intelligence*. Wayne PA: Research Publications.

CHAPTER 6

Therapy Approaches for Patients with Strabismus

One of the most common symptoms exhibited by patients with developmental disabilities, and particularly those with autism, is strabismus. While only about 4 percent of the typical population exhibits strabismus, as many as half of individuals with autism are strabismic.

Strabismus deserves extensive discussion both because of its high prevalence in the special-needs population and because it offers an excellent illustration of the differences in philosophy between developmental optometry and "old school" optometry or ophthalmology. Typically, strabismus is treated surgically by ophthalmologists, creating a cosmetically acceptable eye but doing little to address the underlying cause of the strabismus. Alternately, strabismus resulting in "lazy eye" may be treated by traditional optometrists with eye patches, in order to force the affected eye to work harder.

The developmental optometrist, however, sees strabismus differently. As Brenda Heinke Montecalvo comments, "Strabismus is not an eyeball problem; it is a brain dysfunction for which strabismus is a symptom." In effect, as Montecalvo notes, strabismus is a motor-sensory misalignment caused by the infant's unconscious choice for survival—"an eyeball symptom of a more complicated brain dysfunction."[1] It is of interest that esotropia (strabismus involving an inward turning of the eye) is seen in nearly 7 percent of the population, and yet infants are not born with this condition. Two separate studies, of 1200 and 400 newborns respectively, evaluated the incidence of esotropia in newborns, and found it to be zero. Exotropia, too, typically develops in infancy or early childhood. This is clear evidence that strabismus does not typically stem from structural defects of the eye, but rather is an unconscious adaptive response to neural dysfunction.

This adaptation, in turn, adversely affects a wide range of behaviors. The strabismic individual experiences three basic losses, which are not distinct but overlap. The first is a loss of control of the environment, and of self in relationship to the environment. The second loss is in mobility. The third is a limitation of the range and variety of visual concepts. Strabismic individuals may construct a space, but they will never really perceive space. Perception is a dynamic process by which the human organism obtains information about the immediate environment through the use and integration of sensory receptors, and this cannot occur if the most crucial receptors—the eyes—are not working as a team to perceive three-dimensional space correctly.

We cannot address these problems merely by cosmetically aligning the eyes, which does nothing to retrain the neural system. We can, however, address them quite effectively with therapy.

Over the years, I have treated hundreds of strabismics with great success. Most of these patients' families had been told by doctors that "surgery is the only answer." In reality, however, surgery is *not* the only answer—and, in fact, it is a less optimal treatment approach than therapy, because surgically resectioning the extra-ocular muscles does nothing to influence neural synapses and thus cannot alter behavior and performance in a delayed child. At best, surgeons make patients *appear* more normal, while they continue to suffer from impaired visual processes.

The reliance on surgery to treat strabismus stems from the outdated belief that lost neural synapses cannot regenerate. Newer evidence shows, however, that the synapses of the neuromotor system can indeed do this, and therefore the behaviors and performance associated with constraints of eye movement innervations can be changed. As *New York Times* science journalist John Horgan recently noted, "Indeed, neuroscientists have been repeatedly surprised by the capacity of brain cells to rewire themselves radically, forming new synaptic connections and dissolving old ones, in response to stimulation. Even more surprising is the discovery that adult brains can sprout new cells in a region that underpins the formation of memories." In treating strabismus, what we are seeking is, in Horgan's words, a "self-rewiring" for new adaptive responses—the replacement of

The parents of three-and-a-half-year-old Emily noticed that at times her left eye appeared "lazy" and turned outward. Emily also crawled late, and only for a short period, before she learned to stand and walk. She had delayed speech as well, and bumped into people and objects more often than most toddlers do.

Emily's parents discussed their concerns with her pediatrician, who referred her to a pediatric ophthalmologist. This doctor diagnosed Emily's problem as strabismus and recommended surgery, but her parents came to me for a second opinion.

I told them, "I agree that Emily has an eye movement disorder that can be labeled as a strabismus. However, in my opinion, it is not an organic problem but a functional one, resulting from her developmental disability. I believe it can be solved with vision therapy."

Emily's parents asked, "Why is your opinion different than the ophthalmologist's?" I responded, "Let me show you rather than tell you."

They watched as I had Emily perform the tasks in the Kaplan Nonverbal Battery. A four-ball test indicated right eye suppression, and when I applied yoked base-left prisms she exhibited fusion. When seated and watching television, she tilted her head and body to the left, exhibited poor visual attention, and acted upset. During the balance beam task, she was fearful of getting on the board and had difficulty paying attention; again, the base-left prisms caused a noticeable improvement.

In ball play, Emily displayed a flight reaction. To stimulate her attention, I switched briefly from this task to having Emily walk around the room wearing disruptive prisms, with me holding one hand and her mother holding the other. She was apprehensive at first, but soon relaxed. We returned to the ball play task, and while wearing yoked base-left prisms, Emily was able to catch the ball while standing.

Surprised by the changes they saw in their daughter, Emily's parents opted to try vision therapy. I explained that Emily's response to testing showed that her visual deficits stemmed from problems in orientation, and I prescribed 2-diopter base-left prisms and a program of visual training focusing on the development of body schema.

The results were gratifying: after just four weeks, Emily's parents reported that their daughter's eyes appeared straight almost all of the time. They were thrilled, too, that they'd spared Emily from a surgery that would have traumatized her while at best providing only a cosmetic cure—unlike the real cure that therapy provided.

one form of behavior with another that gives the patient more information in less time, raising the capacity for competent action.

Strabismus is an adaptation precipitated by the conflict between the extra-ocular muscular system and its concomitant, the accommodative muscular system, acting at the same time. To address this problem, we must address its neural roots. When there is a lack of synchronization between what we perceive and our concept of the world, our response is to suppress or diminish perception in an effort to facilitate conception. This leads to a loss of three-dimensional space, and eventually to instability of the visual field.

One strategy that developmentally delayed children with strabismus use to resolve conflicts in intersensory information is to diminish the role of the visual system, and allow the auditory system to dominate. For example, in the Kaplan Nonverbal Battery, the strabismic child will often be seen to listen to the video without watching the picture. Correcting such embedded habits requires more than simply operating on eye muscles, or patching a deviant eye. Doctors who do this leave behind a patient who looks better in family photos, but still suffers from visual impairments that will cause lifelong repercussions.

There are several effective ways to correct strabismus, and the correct method depends upon the individual patient. When treating strabismus, it is important to remember that "one cannot give an erector set to a two-year-old." There is a hierarchical approach that governs visual rehabilitation, and it is important to know where your patient already functions in this hierarchy of skills. As an example, I once treated a family of three strabismics who responded to three different therapy approaches, which I defined based on their ages, level of functioning, and perceptual style. The mother responded to disruptive lenses and procedures incorporating both intrasensory and intersensory feedback. Her strabismus resolved, with resulting reductions in stress and fatigue and improvements in reading ability. Her 14-year-old daughter made great strides in a visual management program aimed at self-orientation and organization, and incorporating activities such as the metronome and Lazy Eight procedures (outlined in later chapters). As a result of therapy, she moved to the top of her class and became active in sports. The second child, a three-year-old, responded well to a home-oriented program including such activities as balloon batting, flashlight tracking with red/green lenses, and a beanbag activity in which she lay on the ground and rolled to touch specified body parts to a beanbag. When she was five, she started a formal visual training program in which she made excellent progress.

Often, as I have discussed earlier, the greatest breakthroughs in therapy for strabismus occur with the use of disruptive lenses, which force a patient to become consciously aware of change. This consciousness causes a startle reaction, which demands an immediate response. This response may move a patient forward or backward in developmental level, and the nature of the reaction will dictate the direction of therapy. For instance, some children react by dropping to the floor and returning to crawling, before moving developmentally upward to a new awareness of self and environment. Other, more emotionally secure patients may manifest a sudden and surprising release, which I refer to as a "breakout" response. Such a response to disruptive yoked prism lenses tends to be much more marked in strabismic patients than in other individuals.

> The reactions of two of my adult strabismic patients provide a good illustration of the "breakout" response to disruptive yoked prism lenses. The first, a 45-year-old psychiatric patient, reacted to disruptive 20-diopter base-down yoked prisms by standing up, dancing about the room, and saying, "This is it! This is how I want to feel." The second patient, a lawyer in her late fifties, initially said when asked to trace a figure eight on the chalkboard, "I can't move the chalk." After I placed 20-diopter base-down yoked prisms on her, she took the chalk and began tracing smooth, flowing lines with abandonment. She asked, "What happened?" I replied, "I just took the ropes off you."

Another simple procedure used in my office is particularly effective in treating strabismic children who "tune out" visual information and rely instead on auditory stimuli. The procedure involves the use of a metronome and a vectograph, which is an illuminated plastic holder with two separate images placed at the top and bottom. The patient, wearing polaroid lenses, is asked to look first at the top image (which requires the two eyes to be viewing in parallel) and then at the bottom figure (which requires the eyes to be converged to keep the figures fused), moving the eyes at each beat of the metronome. When fusion occurs, the patient will see the bottom figure "floating" forward in the air. Often a younger patient will swipe at the figure in the air in an attempt to feel it, trusting the sense of touch more than the sense of sight. This procedure causes a recalibration of the binocular neural cells, leading to ocular alignment, which is consolidated through training.

A.J. Kirscher, an optometrist in Montreal, called me one day and said, "Mel, I have a patient in Toronto who is a topographer by trade but needs to hire someone to read the maps because he can't see the depth. I think you could help him."

The gentleman showed up at my office after a 12-hour train trip. Following my evaluation, I prescribed yoked base-up prisms for a centering problem. I placed a pair of 5-diopter yoked base-up prisms on him, and asked him to sit down in front of the vectograph with polaroids over the yoked prisms. I set the metronome to 48 beats per minute and told him not to worry about what he saw, but simply to move his eyes from one image to the other in time to the beat.

In less than one minute, the man became aware that the object appeared to be floating in space, an indication that he was seeing in depth. He turned to me and said, "It was worth the trip."

In correcting strabismus in children with autism spectrum disorders or other developmental disabilities, the question arises: should patching be employed? Developmental optometrists who use patching recognize that for the child it is both scary and frustrating, and that children's negative reactions limit the amount of time that patches can be used.

I have chosen to avoid patching in my approach to treating any visual anomaly, whether strabismus or amblyopia, because normal binocular function in early development requires synchronized input from both of a child's eyes. Physiologists David Hubel and Torsten Wiesel, who won a Nobel Prize for their work on visual input to the brain, concluded that occluding (patching) will gradually lead to the disappearance of visual cells that respond to both eyes simultaneously, eventually leading a child to pay attention to the input of only one eye at a time.

My preference for eliminating the suppression resulting from diplopia in children is to stimulate eye movement coordination by creating binocular diplopia, which overrides the need for suppression—the reason for the eye turning in the first place.

My procedure is to have the child seated with red/green anaglyph (3-D) glasses behind 20-diopter prisms, with the right lens in the base-up position and the left lens in the base-down position. A ball is hung at chest level, 36 inches in front of the child, and the child is asked to follow the ball's movements. The verbal child will tell you that he or she sees two balls: one red, the other green. The nonverbal child will be asked to point at red and then green. Sometimes when I cannot elicit a response, I give the child a stick and say, "Try to hit the ball." The child may hit the "red ball" or swing at the space above or below.

Michael Brenner is proof that surgery and patching do not remediate the neural deficits underlying strabismus, while prism lenses and vision therapy can. His mother describes the family's experiences with surgery and patching, and Michael's reaction to prism lenses:

My son was born four and a half years ago with significant optic nerve atrophy and strabismus (crossed eyes). At 18 months Michael wore a patch over one eye in order to help his strabismus. By 19 months he was operated on for his muscle weakness. Although the surgery appeared to be a success, Michael never seemed to see normally. He would tilt his head while reading a book or watching TV, and he didn't appear to notice me until I was in close proximity. Conversely, his peripheral vision was excellent. He was able to visually track, although it was quite selective. Even though two ophthalmologists felt that Michael's optic nerve damage altered his vision somewhat, neither doctor thought that glasses were necessary at the time. After meeting with Dr. Kaplan, I was quite certain that Michael had a visual-spatial problem and could be helped. I was right.

My son has only been wearing the prism glasses for six weeks, but the benefits have been incredible and very encouraging. I immediately saw a drastic improvement in Michael's gait: he seldom toe-walks, and his feet rarely turn in anymore. His teachers have noticed increased attention and verbalization, which we have also seen at home. Michael's receptive language has also improved, and we've actually had a few small "conversations." Prior to wearing prism glasses, Michael had poor eye contact. Now, he occasionally looks right at me—not through me... My once passive son not only plays with toys now, but actually competes with his assertive sister for them.

With therapy, we were able to consolidate these gains, allowing Michael to perform at a far higher level than his doctors had earlier predicted. Surgery had made Michael's eyes *appear* normal; but prism lenses and therapy made them *work* normally with his brain. The result was significant improvement not just in overt visual processes such as eye contact, but also in communication, socialization, and other behaviors that many parents or professionals would assume had nothing to do with vision.

The goal is not to change the anatomical projection from retina to visual cortex, but rather to create a recoding of a new visual spatial framework. This causes the patient's mind to recognize the difference between the new and old models by virtue of what the eyes see and the feeling of the movement. As researchers I.P. Howard and W.B. Templeton note, "Where there is a rapid adaptation of movement to distorted vision, over distances far greater than the normal range of error of those movements, an initial stage of gross inhibition of old habits and the substitutions of new responses must occur."

Such procedures facilitate the development of normal neural pathways, rather than suppressing them as patching or surgery may. Thus, therapy leads to higher visual performance, while patching or surgery do not improve and may actually further impair visual processes.

It is natural for parents to focus solely on improving the cosmetic appearance of an eye that turns in or out, and to select the instant "cure" of surgery or the inexpensive "cure" of patching as a result, because few parents are aware that strabismus is not a core problem in itself but rather a response to neural dysfunction. Clinicians need to help these parents understand that unlike surgery, vision training can treat this underlying dysfunction—and unlike patching, therapy can remediate neural deficits rather than running the risk of creating new ones.

Note

1   Montecalvo, B. (2000) "Infant and toddler strabismus and amblyopia." *Behavioural Aspects of Vision Care 41*, 2, 16–20.

CHAPTER 7

Therapy Approaches for Patients with Orientation Issues

The most dramatic stage in early cognitive development occurs when an infant realizes for the first time that there is "me" and "not me." This awareness of the physical self, or body schema, forms the basis for all future exploration and understanding of the outside world. As scientist Gerd Sommerhoff notes, "Since the body functions as an important frame of reference in the perception of spatial relations, the brain's internal representations of the external world can be complete only to the extent to which they are integrated with the internal representation of body posture and movement."[1]

When an individual cannot create an accurate body schema, he or she is also incapable of creating an accurate picture of external space. Thus, the saying, "As we are, so is our world," is true in a biological as well as a philosophical sense. Our perception of objects in our environment—how large or small they are, how near or close, even how they feel when touched—depends in large part on our knowledge of our bodies' physical limits, the positions of our limbs, and our position in relation to space.

An interesting example of this is "Alice in Wonderland" syndrome, a very rare and temporary consequence of migraines, Epstein-Barr infection, or epilepsy. Individuals affected by this syndrome (which may stem from altered blood flow to cortical areas containing the "mental map" of the body) experience a dramatically altered body image, and can no longer correctly sense their own size and shape. As a consequence, they feel as if they have grown to gigantic proportions or, conversely, as if they have shrunk to a tiny size. At the same time objects around them also appear altered in size or distance, with automobiles looking like toy cars or the ground appearing far closer than it really is, and objects feel odd or unpleasant when touched.

These symptoms are terrifying, but fortunately quite temporary. The same is not true, however, for the patients I treat for problems in orientation. In their cases, innate neural deficits cause a chronic distortion of body schema. For them, confusion is not a temporary condition but a way of life. They have no clear concept of where their bodies end and the outer world begins. They have trouble sensing the position of their arms, legs, hands, feet, and head. They lack the ability to imitate, a skill that is crucial to learning. Their inner distortion leads to a distorted sense of their surroundings, making the outside world seem unpredictable and frightening. To help these patients, we must first rehabilitate their body schema, which will often lead to remediation of impairments in spatial organization as well.

My clinical experience has shown that internal constraints lead to environmental constraints, and therapy for orientation issues must address both. In designing a visual management program for patients with impairments in body schema, it is important to follow a developmental sequence from postural awareness to movement awareness to hearing and moving, and then to hearing, seeing, and moving. Here are procedures appropriate for each stage:

- *Stage 1 (postural awareness):* Procedures that focus on attention to postural reflexes involved in control of body attitude and the position of body parts in relation to each other—for example, rolling on the floor, jumping on a trampoline, using a balance board.

- *Stage 2 (movement awareness):* Procedures that focus on the role of internal proprioceptive control of the limbs in relation to posture. In general, procedures should progress from seated to standing, and should move from control of individual body parts to control of same-side limbs (e.g., right leg and right arm) and then opposite-side limbs (e.g., right leg and left arm). Sample procedures include Angels, Simon Says, and the Dowel Guide procedure outlined below.

Seated dowel procedure

This is an extraordinarily effective procedure that can be tailored to the developmental level of your patient. It incorporates movement, awareness, and crossing of the midline of the body, and is an excellent way to address body schema. As I will discuss in Chapter 9, it also aids in creating respiratory synergies in patients whose dysfunctional breathing patterns contribute to anxiety and vision problems.

Necessary materials include a 3-foot-long dowel with a 1-inch diameter, a mirror, and two chairs.

Procedure

Ask your patient to sit facing you, with a mirror positioned so the patient can see his or her reflection. The patient should be able to see his or her entire body in the mirror, and the therapist's body should be slightly to one side to avoid blocking the patient's view of the mirror.

The patient should grasp the dowel with two hands, palms facing down. Place your hands in between the patient's, in the center of the dowel. Then guide the patient in the following movements, taking care to observe the patient's visual attention, breathing, and coordination and control. Encourage the patient to attend to his or her reflection in the mirror throughout the exercise.

Initially the patient should hold the dowel with arms fully extended at the middle section of the body. This is the patient's "midpoint." All movements should begin and end at this point.

The first movement that the patient will execute, with your guidance, is "up." The patient should pull in a deep breath and (if verbal) say the word "up." The patient should bring the dowel in a smooth, even motion above the head until the arms are fully extended over the head, while breathing out in a relaxed and complete manner. Your hands should remain in the center of the dowel in order to guide the patient in this movement. The patient should then return the dowel to the midpoint while breathing in. These movements should be smooth, controlled, *and slow. The breath in and out should be full and complete.*

The next direction is down. The patient (if verbal) should say the word "down" and then breathe out while bringing the dowel down to the knees in a slow, smooth, and controlled manner. Once the patient has lowered the dowel, guide the patient to pause briefly, and then bring the dowel back to the midpoint while pulling the breath back in. The patient's breathing and movement should be as outlined above.

The next direction is right. The patient, if verbal, should say the word "right." Guide the patient in bringing the dowel in a smooth horizontal plane to the patient's complete right as the patient breathes out. The patient should then return the dowel to the midpoint with your assistance, while breathing in. The breathing should again be smooth, slow and complete.

The last direction in which the patient needs to move the dowel is left. The patient, if verbal, should say the word "left" and then, with your guidance, bring the dowel to the complete left while breathing out. The patient should then bring the dowel back to the midpoint while breathing in.

This exercise should be practiced for approximately five minutes.

Standing dowel procedure

This is a variant of the seated dowel procedure outlined above. Necessary materials include a 3-foot-long dowel with a 1-inch diameter, and a full-length mirror hung vertically. The procedure for this exercise is the same as outlined above, except the patient stands facing the mirror and the trainer faces the patient. The trainer should stand slightly to the side of the patient so as to not block the patient's image in the mirror.

- *Stage 3 (sensory integration of auditory and proprioceptive cues):*
  Procedures that begin the process of integrating internal and external processes. For example, set a metronome to 48 beats per minute and have your patient perform the same procedures as in Stage 2, but this time to the beat of the metronome. A note: some patients with a global style prefer to self-initiate rather than being directed by the metronome, and in these cases I start with music to integrate hearing and movement.

- *Stage 4 (sensory integration/orchestration):* Procedures that focus on integrating three sensory modalities. For an example, see the "Checkerboard Marching" procedure that follows.

Checkerboard Marching with metronome

Checkerboard Materials

Metronome or tape of metronome

Procedure

PART I: Place the checkerboard at the patient's eye level and ask the patient to stand in front of it. Turn on the metronome tape or set the metronome to 48 beats per minute.

Instruct the patient to use the left index finger to touch the first orange box in the top row. As the patient touches the orange box, he or she should also raise the left leg in front of the body, bending it at the knee. This should be done on the first beat of the metronome.

The patient should then lower the arm and touch his or her side at the same time that the leg is lowered. This movement should be done on the second beat. The patient should next be instructed to lift the right finger to touch the last orange box in the first row, while lifting the right leg by bending it at the knee. This is done on the third beat. The patient should then lower the arm, touching his or her side, and the leg, on the fourth beat.

The patient should be instructed to go on to the second row using the same pattern, touching the first orange box with the left finger while raising the left leg, lowering the arm and leg, then touching the last orange box with the right finger while raising the right leg, and then lowering it.

Each movement should be done in time to the beat of the metronome. The patient should continue in this manner for the remainder of the chart.

PART II: Ask the patient to repeat Part I, but this time, have the patient lift the *left* arm and *right* leg together, and then the *right* arm and *left* leg together. For example, the patient will touch the first orange box in the row with his or her *left* finger, while lifting the *right* leg, in time to the beat of the metronome. The arm and leg should then be lowered, on the beat, and then the patient should touch the last orange box in the row with his or her *right* finger, while lifting the *left* leg, on the beat. The limbs should then be lowered, on the beat.

Throughout Parts I and II the trainer should be aware of the patient's visual attention to the task, the accuracy of the patient's tracking, the coordination of his or her movements, and his or her ability to stay on the beat.

While the four developmental stages I've outlined should typically be addressed in the order given, the procedures you select should vary according to your patients' abilities and needs. As the following cases illustrate, deficits in orientation affect patients in different ways depending on their age, level of development, intellectual ability, and perceptual style. Thus, the clinician needs to be flexible in creating a program that is most effective in putting each patient "back on track" developmentally.

Some case studies

Tory: A little girl who wouldn't leave the house

Tory was five years old, and her mother was concerned about her physical, social, and emotional well-being. She was a toe-walker, didn't like to go outside and play with other children, and was easily startled by noise or moving objects. Tory told her mother once, "My brain doesn't work well. Why don't we take it out and wash it off, and put it back?"

My analysis of Tory indicated that her eyes were free of pathology. She had 20/20 acuity, and ocular fusion was present. During the Kaplan Nonverbal Battery, she was fearful on the balance board while watching television. She had difficulty balancing on one foot, and displayed a midline problem when doing floor angels. She was unable to time the ball during standing ball play, but improved when she was seated. When she walked to and from a mirror, she had to turn to see where she was going.

Tory responded positively to yoked base-up prisms during visual tasks, but her orientation difficulties persisted. I recommended a program of visual management, and a prescription of plano 1-degree base-up yoked prisms for full-time wear.

Tory had a global perceptual style but her behavior was focal, her space-world was tunneled, and her impaired orientation to gravity caused her to be fearful. Although children's postural reflexes are innate, these reflexes are quite primitive and must be developed over time. As a result of Tory's developmental delays, this maturation of postural reflexes had not occurred.

I told Tory's mother, "We cannot put Tory back in the crib, but we can establish a playing field where she can experiment with these reflexes." The procedures I designed for Tory began with her seated and then progressed to standing, so that she could isolate her spatial cues prior to integrating them with her proprioceptive movements.

The first stage of Tory's program involved mirror fusion, progressing from seated to standing to walking. In this way we allowed Tory to deal with her visual system in isolation, before adding gravitational demands and then movement.

In the second phase of Tory's therapy, I used disruptive yoked prism lenses to induce a spatial rearrangement of her space-world in sitting, standing, and walking conditions. The light transformation of the prisms awakened her nervous system, causing her to attend to her global world. (This is similar to auditory training, in which autistic children who have reduced their attention to auditory frequencies are bombarded by a full range of frequencies.) A full range of light-ray frequencies signalled Tory to be "awake," and to attend to movement and depth.

As she progressed to standing and moving while wearing disruptive prisms, Tory needed to learn to distribute her energy between visual and vestibular cues, and to orchestrate seeing, hearing and moving. To help her do this, I used a combination of directive and disruptive procedures. These procedures, and the spatial illusions created by the yoked prism lenses, were enough to put Tory back on a path of sequential and orderly development. In three months' time, her mother reported that it was difficult to get Tory in the house because she had so many friends and sports activities. Her toe-walking had virtually disappeared as well.

Joe: A loss of stability of visual judgment

Tory, the patient in the previous example, was a child with minor problems, which at worst could be classified as pathological shyness and fearfulness.

However, similar therapy approaches also are highly effective for patients with more severe disabilities. One of these patients was Joe, a nonverbal eight-year-old whose symptoms were consistent with autism spectrum disorder.

Joe exhibited a range of "stims," avoided ball sports, and still needed training wheels on his bicycle. When he walked down a hallway, he had to glide his hand along the face of the wall in order to know where he was.

A matching test concluded that Joe had 20/30 visual acuity and no eye pathology. The Kaplan Nonverbal Battery, however, was much more informative. During seated and standing eye tracking procedures, Joe's eyes failed to follow. When I tried yoked base-up prisms with a bell added to provide auditory input, he made some attempt to track. When I added proprioception, his performance moved to a higher level. This indicated that Joe's neuromuscular complex lacked the lower-level synergies needed for natural and automatic movement, forcing higher-level neurological processes to participate in the process. This forced Joe to use excess energy to perform simple tasks.

During the seated television task, Joe locked his feet around the chair, ignored the television visually while paying attention to auditory stimuli, and increased his inappropriate body movements. In standing ball play, yoked prism lenses made no difference. When he performed this task seated, with 5-diopter base-up yoked prisms, I detected increased visual attention and performance in both the balloon and the ball task. His postural reflexes in response to the television or a mirror indicated delays in body awareness and control.

From Joe's actions during testing, I learned that he lacked appropriate eye movement of sufficient magnitude during movement, indicating a lack of integration of central and peripheral visual clues. He was unaware of the feeling of his eye movements and didn't trust the spatial feedback from his environment. His impaired optokinetic reflex—the reflex that causes intermittent rotation of the eye while looking at moving objects, in order to compensate for body and head movements so the movement of the retinal image is minimized—inhibited his ability to project his body coordinates to match his environmental coordinates.

My test results gave me the direction I needed in order to plan Joe's therapy. My goals were, first, to establish postural reflexes, second, to stabilize Joe's visual field, and third, to stabilize the relationships between Joe's eye movements, head, and posture. One procedure I used was Lazy

Eight and Lazy Eight with Disruptives (see below), which facilitates eye tracking and proprioceptive interaction.

Lazy Eight standing

Materials

1 large chalkboard
½-inch diameter chalk

Procedure

Hang the chalkboard horizontally on the wall in front of the patient so that the center of the chalkboard is at the eye level of the patient. Draw a large sideways 8 on the chalkboard. It should be approximately 2 feet across. Give the patient a piece of chalk to hold. The chalk should be held in the patient's dominant hand.

Direct the patient to trace the sideways 8. Observe the patient's visual attention and attention to task. The patient should trace the form approximately 30 times with the dominant hand and then repeat with the other hand.

Observe the patient's movement. Throughout the procedure, did the patient cross the midline of the sideways 8? Did the patient continuously move the chalk in a smooth, even manner? Observe the patient's breathing and stress level throughout the procedure.

Lazy Eight standing with Disruption

Materials

1 large chalkboard
chalk
1 pair 15- or 20-degree adjustable prisms

Procedure

Follow the procedure described above, with the addition of the disruptive lenses. If the patient currently wears a prescription to correct acuity, place the disruptive prisms over the patient's own glasses.

Observe the patient's movement as before. If your patient has correctly reorganized his or her spatial perception with the aid of the disruptive prisms, he or she should describe the bottom of the figure

8 as appearing closer if wearing base-up disruptive prisms, and the top of the figure as appearing closer if wearing base-down. When the prisms are placed in the base-left position, the right side of the 8 should appear closer; when the prisms are placed in the base-right position, the left side should appear closer.

In some cases, patients will see partial change or their visual attention to figure/ground will be incomplete and different planes will appear closer. The response to what the patient "sees" will usually occur prior to what the patient "feels."

As your patient starts to attend to spatial rearrangement changes, you will see a more erect posture, relaxation of the body, and a more flowing movement of the arm. The synergistic action of the neuromotor system is uniting a greater number of synapses at this stage, and as a result the patient sees and feels more in less time, leaving more time for thinking.

Joe responded well to these procedures. In three months' time, he was riding a two-wheel bike without training wheels, and he no longer needed to trail his hand across the wall when walking down a corridor. In six months, he added 20 words to his vocabulary.

These changes appeared to stem largely from an improved sense of gravity. Initially, Joe's neuromotor constraints made it impossible for him to meet the demands associated with vertical posture and movement. When he developed new synergies with the help of prism lenses and therapy, his improved sense of gravity improved his posture, his ability to move comfortably, his sense of security, and his ability to move his eyes efficiently in a vertical as well as a horizontal direction.

Noah: Reversing the feedback loop

When Noah, a 6-foot-tall, 21-year-old man with autism, started vision therapy, he exhibited severe problems in orientation. I began with tasks designed to make Noah aware of the movement of his own body and, by extension, allow him to develop a body schema.

One of these was a simple exercise involving a dowel. Initially, I guided the dowel while Noah held it passively. Next, I asked Noah to imitate my movements, while he held the dowel independently. The third step required Noah to initiate movements on his own, using the dowel as an aid.

Noah was able to accomplish these tasks readily, so we moved to a higher level of demand. This time, I asked Noah to move his limbs without using the dowel as a crutch to help him determine the orientation of his body. I found that he could respond correctly when I asked him to touch my hand with his right or left hand. Also, he could raise his right foot and touch my hand with the point of the foot. When asked to raise his right hand and right foot simultaneously, however, he could not perform the movement.

My question was: Is this a hardware or a software problem? Most doctors would attribute Noah's problem to a structural defect of the sensory cortex, but I concluded that since Noah could control his limbs in the earlier exercises, it was a software issue and thus amenable to therapy.

I tried moving both of Noah's limbs to guide him, but with no success. Next, I tried letting him watch himself in the mirror, but he still did not make any progress. From my readings in neurology, I'd learned of the concept of muscle potentiation, in which afferent movement from the brain can stimulate movement of a limb—an alternative to oculomotor recalibration. When a feed-forward loop doesn't work, movement from the limbs can sometimes stimulate neural awareness and re-establish neural control of the feed-forward/feedback loop of limb movement. This sounded like a promising approach.

I sat Noah in a chair and tied a cord around his right foot, tying the other end of the cord around his right hand. I then asked Noah to raise his right hand and touch my hand, which caused the hand to pull his right leg up. After a few rehearsals, Noah was able to raise his arm and leg on command. Over time, he moved from needing my guidance to initiating this movement on his own. The next step was to remove the cord and repeat the task. This time, Noah was able to simultaneously move his right leg and right hand, and also could simultaneously move his left leg and right hand.

A more remarkable development occurred when I asked Noah to stand next to me in front of the mirror and imitate my movements as he watched my reflection. I said, "Noah, as you raise your arm and leg, say, 'one.'" He responded by saying, "One," and moving correctly. We kept moving and counting out loud, until we reached "Ten." Next, I asked Noah to move and count by himself. He did, but then he suddenly stopped and began to count, over and over and very quickly, "One-two-three-four-five-six-seven-eight-nine-ten." I finally had to intervene to get him to stop.

At the time I was working with a developmental pediatrician, Lillian Ko. Dr. Ko found Noah's response fascinating, saying that it was typical of a two-and-a-half-year-old child. The simple exercises Noah had performed had awakened formerly dormant neural processes in his brain, causing this nonverbal man to reach a level of development he had failed to achieve in his earliest years of childhood.

Eric: The importance of sensory "grounding"

Eric, the four-year-old son of a physician, came to my office after receiving a diagnosis of pervasive developmental disorder and perceptual developmental delay. His occupational therapist recommended that his parents seek my help, and they reluctantly agreed.

Eric displayed the typical characteristics of a child with PDD: he was nonverbal, socially isolated, and hyperactive. He also held his head tilted at an angle. He was able to follow directions, and responded positively to yoked base-up and yoked base-left prisms when watching television. During the rocking board activity he reacted more positively to base-left than to base-up yoked prisms. He also responded well to base-left yoked prisms during the standing pursuits task, but less well during seated pursuits. In the ball play task, he performed best with yoked base-up prisms while standing, but with yoked base-left prisms while seated. His eye movements were fair.

Eric's responsiveness to prism lenses during testing encouraged me to offer a positive prognosis. Eric's father told me that his chief goal for the boy was to develop language, which I believed could happen within four to six months. A second goal was for Eric to ride a bike, which I predicted would occur earlier. The third goal we set was that Eric's social abilities would improve.

The first question I addressed in planning Eric's vision therapy was whether his training should be directed toward orientation or organization. I chose to focus initially on relieving Eric's constraints in orientation. These constraints limited the time and energy Eric had free to attend to visual cues, causing him to constrict his peripheral vision and forcing him to make excessive eye movements. They also caused his hyperactivity, which was a survival mechanism he used to establish the limits of "self." I prescribed yoked base-left prisms, with the understanding that when Eric's self-induced constraints in orientation were reduced, the lenses would be changed to yoked base-up lenses to improve his timing in spatial actions.

I began with simple procedures such as having Eric stand on the rocking board while watching television. I did not ask Eric to perform in front of a mirror at first, because the results of my testing told me that he would be overwhelmed if his initial therapy required him to pay too much attention to self.

In my experience, people with global perceptual styles are more relaxed when they do not need to attend to cues involving orientation. Their behavior is driven by the survival instinct, and they lock onto objects in space with such intensity that they lose awareness of self when standing. Their eye movements appear smoother but their inner tension increases due to loss of attention to self. (I had one long-term psychiatric patient tell me that he needed the tension within him in order to function, because otherwise he had no awareness of "self" in space.) In these cases, when patients are seated, the chair gives them support and they can feel their bodies. This results in a relaxed posture and reduced attention to space, resulting in increased saccadic eye movements.

The plan, in such cases, is to ground the patient in some sensory system, freeing up the visual system for a relaxed exploration of the environment. With younger patients such as Eric, I start with antigravity procedures to create posture awareness; these include balance board rocking and rocking on the floor. Movement awareness exercises include the dowel procedures, "angels," standing and marching (progressing from individual limbs to same-side limbs to opposite-side limbs), standing and marching, and "walk and sit" with disruptive glasses. To integrate auditory processes, we have patients clap or march in time to music or the metronome. Finally, we add the checkerboard procedure outlined earlier. When this is accomplished, we implement procedures such as bunting a ball, to improve timing and the centering of visual processing.

In Eric's case it took two months to re-establish a body schema, and two additional months to establish an intersensory coordination between his visual and vestibular systems. The procedures I used followed a developmental sequence, from postural awareness to movement awareness, to hearing and moving, then hearing, seeing, and moving.

My predictions were right on schedule: in five months, Eric was producing three- to four-word phrases. His orientation improved markedly, and he began testing his parents with his discovery of his self-image. Many of his PDD symptoms became less obvious, or disappeared altogether.

Does this change in performance and adaptation mean that Eric no longer has PDD? I can't answer that question. My goal is not to worry about diagnostic categories, but to reduce Eric's symptoms and raise his level of performance. This will enhance his learning, reduce his stress, and allow him to interact socially with his world. As long as he continues to make excellent progress on these fronts, I am happy to leave the labels to others.

Tim: A case of "toeing in"

Many autistic children toe in when they walk, making their gait odd and clumsy. This behavior is not innate but learned, and results from orientation problems.

Tim, a six-year-old autistic child, toed in his left foot when walking, but held his feet straight when standing. He was nonverbal, and exhibited motor delays in both general and specific body movements. He was unable to blow out candles, had problems with eye contact, and had a fetish for letters and numbers. (In fact, when he entered the vision therapy room, he noticed a board with magnetic letters, rushed to it, and started to play with the letters. Neither his parents nor I could divert his attention and get him back on task.)

During the Kaplan Nonverbal Battery, Tim responded positively to yoked base-left prisms. When I placed these lenses on him, his posture improved when seated, his standing balance improved, and he reacted more positively to ball play.

I have been prescribing directive yoked prisms for many years for patients who routinely toe in. In time, the spatial rearrangement of the lenses leads to a reorientation of the body and a substitution of new habits for old ones. Once this consolidation occurs, the prisms can be removed and the new posture remains. However, children on the autism spectrum have moved away from trusting their visual systems, and tend to be insensitive to the use of directive lenses to reduce toeing in. Therefore, to stimulate a response to spatial rearrangement, it is often necessary to employ disruptive yoked prisms in magnitudes of 15 to 20 diopters. This rotation of the optical array causes a startled, conscious awareness, and a need for redeployment of both visual and kinesthetic attention. In some cases it creates fear, while in others it creates relief.

To sustain the attention that the disruptive prisms create, it is necessary to follow with procedures that are familiar to the patient. This gives the patient time to create new "movement memory"—that is, to develop memories of the new "feel" of doing familiar actions in a different way. The use of disruptive yoked prisms to create rapid conscious change, followed by full-time wearing of directive yoked prisms, leads to a consolidation of new motor planning.

In Tim's case, disruptive yoked prisms caused signs of relief and an obvious sense of freedom. It was as if he'd been visually tied up, and now was free. When I put 20-diopter base-down yoked prisms on him, he walked around the room and inspected everything. His posture was straight, but he still toed in. When I switched to 20-diopter base-left lenses, he walked without toeing in. Each time I reached out to take the disruptive lenses off, he would try to get them back. Instead, I gave him a pair of 5-diopter yoked base-left prisms housed in the same frame. While wearing them, he walked with his feet straight.

Tim's therapy included movement procedures such as side-to-side and forward-and-backward rocking on the balance board. The side-to-side rocking gave Tim neural information as to where he was in space, and the forward-and-backward rocking gave him information about where other objects were. I also implemented specific motor planning procedures such as ball bunting (first seated and then standing) and rail-walking while watching himself in a mirror. At this point, Tim was wearing 2-diopter base-left yoked prisms, and his gait was straight. I moved him to procedures focusing on spatial organization, and changed his prescription to 2-diopter base-up prisms.

Tim continued to establish postural awareness and laterality, with his toeing in decreasing as a result. As his constraints diminished, he began to enjoy his new freedom of movement, and eventually he exhibited increases in vocabulary.

Expanding our view of optometry

I'm sometimes asked by more traditional vision professionals if the procedures I use to address orientation issues, such as those I've outlined in this chapter, really qualify as optometry. My answer is that "anything visual is optometry"—and who is better able to help these patients than an optometrist? My criterion, quite simply, is that therapy must result in a patient with better visual skills. The patients I've described in this chapter all improved greatly in response to therapy designed to ameliorate deficits in orientation. This is only logical, because we cannot fully understand and interact with our world—visually or in any other way—until we understand our place in it.

Improvements in body schema and orientation allow patients to answer the crucial question, "Where am I?" This results in a remarkable change in how these patients see themselves in relation to their world, and as a result in how they feel, behave, and learn. In lower-functioning patients you will often see improvements including better gait and posture, improved coordination, fewer "stims," reduced self-injury, a reduction in anxiety and fears, a greater ability to learn by imitation, a happier mood, increased verbalization, and more self-confidence. In higher-functioning patients, you will typically see physical and emotional changes as well as progress in higher-level cognitive skills, career and sports performance, and interpersonal relationships.

In short, when you enable your patients to develop a better sense of "self," you will elevate them to a new stage of awareness that is a prerequisite for a higher level of both visual and overall performance—and that is the highest goal of developmental optometry.

Note

1   Sommerhoff, G. Cited by Beck, A. (2000) in "Cognitive mapping and radio drama." *Consciousness, Literature and the Arts 1*, 2.

CHAPTER 8

Therapy Approaches for Patients with Spatial Organization Issues

Children and adults with impaired spatial organization skills live in a world where perception and reality constantly clash, and nothing is truly where it seems to be. Their inability to accurately interpret or predict events around them makes them tense, anxious, and fearful. Many are clumsy, falling frequently or bumping into other people accidentally. Some can't hit a baseball, while others have trouble even buttoning a shirt or eating with a knife and fork. Many can't read well, because it's hard to locate the words on the page. For higher-functioning people with spatial organization deficits, driving is a white-knuckle experience and navigating a crowded street can be stress-provoking. For those with more obvious problems, even the simplest activities—sitting in a classroom, swinging on the playground, watching television—can provoke extreme anxiety.

The more significant the conflict between spatial perception and reality, the more severe the resulting symptoms will be. In children with autism, for example, severe impairments in spatial organization contribute to aloofness and poor social skills (because people are alarming or incomprehensible if you cannot predict their actions); gait problems (because you can't move easily if you misperceive the floor, walls, and objects around you); and hyperactivity (because when your visual sense can't comprehend your environment, you will replace it with touch and movement). Other symptoms we frequently see in autistic or non-autistic patients with spatial organization deficits include anxiety or panic attacks, learning disabilities, and significant impairments in coordination.

To cope with the perceptual conflicts cause by spatial organization impairment, many patients develop habits that constrain their visual system, such as strabismus, over-reliance on auditory or other non-visual stimuli, or "tunnel vision." These constraints, in turn, have far-reaching effects on their ability to learn, communicate, and respond normally to their world. When therapy succeeds in removing these constraints, we often see corresponding gains both in vision and in social, academic, and communication skills, as the following case studies will illustrate.

Some case studies

Jenny: A breakthrough in communicative skills

Jenny, a five-year-old nonverbal autistic child, was apprehensive during testing and displayed a global perceptual style with fast-moving saccadic eye tracking. Like many patients with autism spectrum disorders, she lacked the ability to sustain continuous movements of her eyes when following an object, resulting in retinal instability and poor perception. Jenny displayed severe problems in both spatial orientation and spatial organization. Her best visual acuity based on the Kindergarten Matching Test was 20/100, probably as a result of her lateral nystagmus. She performed better seated than standing, and responded best to yoked base-up prisms.

I prescribed plano 2-diopter base-up yoked prisms, and told Jenny's parents to return in one month for visual management therapy. The first goal for Jenny was to create awareness of the space around her, through the use of the prisms and basic therapy activities.

When Jenny returned to my office, her parents reported positive changes in her posture as a result of the yoked lenses. However, she still appeared apprehensive. In planning her therapy, I took her fears into account. To maximize her motivation, while addressing her visual deficits, I based her visual management program on the following concepts:

- The level of demand would be at or below her level of ability, ensuring success.

- The program would start with Jenny's strengths, and move to her weaknesses. As she succeeded, her fears would decrease, and she would become more open to challenging tasks.

- Activities would offer both novelty and reward.

- Activities would be dynamic, not static.

My choice, in selecting an initial task, was to have Jenny bunt a ball while seated. This is a global-style task that requires vergent eye movements, and provides both novelty and a high chance of success. Jenny worked through five variations of this task:

1. bunting a 9-inch balloon with a pizza tin

2. bunting a 9-inch balloon with a rolling pin

3. bunting a 2½-inch ball with a pizza tin

4. bunting a 2½-inch ball with a rolling pin

5. catching the ball.

This task was structured to move from a very simple stage to more difficult stages, and the pizza tin provided novelty and reinforcement because Jenny enjoyed the noise it made when she hit the ball with it. By the time we reached the last stage, Jenny was relaxed, she reached out easily to catch the ball, and she smiled happily when she succeeded. She had reached a new level of perception, and found it highly rewarding.

Jenny's changes in performance and emotional state were so dramatic that I decided to see if the experience had made an impact on her visual acuity. As I've noted earlier, patients with nystagmus sometimes demonstrate a very sudden and marked improvement following the use of yoked prism lenses and training.

I ushered Jenny, now calm and relaxed, into the exam room. Using the same kindergarten chart, I pointed to a figure and again asked Jenny to select a card with the same figure. She succeeded on the 20/100 line, just as before in testing. Next, she succeeded in identifying figures on the 20/80 line. When I showed her a heart on the 20/50 line, her parents and I were shocked to hear this nonverbal little girl say, "Heart." On the same line I isolated a circle, and again she responded correctly with "Circle," We continued, and she spoke the names of all of the figures on the same line.

Vision expert Alfred Yarbus once stated, "The first limitation to perceptual and conceptual development is physiological and subject to change." As Jenny's unexpected verbalization in response to vision therapy shows, this change, when it occurs, can be remarkable and nearly instantaneous.

Teddy: A sensory awakening

Four-year-old Teddy loved television, but he only wanted to watch the credits of the Barney cartoon his parents brought to my office. He listened rather than looked at the picture until the credits started to roll, and would rewind the tape so he could watch the credits over and over. He liked to watch spinning objects, had a fetish for numbers and letters, and avoided situations that required eye movement and depth perception. Based on this and other observations, I prescribed 3-diopter base-down yoked prisms for Teddy, and recommended vision therapy to help him use his senses in an integrated way.

Teddy displayed delays in orientation and motor planning, as well as delays in spatial organization. Since survival for Teddy meant attention to self rather than his spatial environment, I decided to begin his therapy with orientation and motor planning, then integrate his movement and auditory processes, and finally build on these neural awakenings to integrate visual attention. This would allow Teddy to move from fixational eye movements to saccadic eye movements, and to develop a spatial awareness of figure/ground.

In one activity, I sat across from Teddy, raised my arm, and then brought it down to touch my knee. After a few repetitions, I took Teddy's hand, raising it and then releasing it so it fell and touched his knee. Next, I set a metronome at 48 beats per minute. I raised my hand and stopped at the first beat, and then lowered my hand so it touched my knee on the second beat. I repeated this move several times, and then physically guided Teddy to raise his hand on the first beat and lower it on the second beat. Gradually, I faded my prompt and Teddy learned to raise his hand to touch mine on the first beat; I would hold his hand briefly, so that when he lowered it, his timing matched the second beat. Once he began to feel the beat, I moved my own hand up and down, allowing him to initiate his movements independently. When I stopped, he continued the action.

Over time, Teddy learned to move his right or left hand up and down to the beat, and then to alternate side-to-side (right hand to left knee and vice versa). He then moved on to performing this activity while standing.

Next, it was time to add a visual component by placing numbers in a single line, and asking Teddy to touch the numbers in sequence (from 1 to 2 and back again, repeating the procedure). I guided him through this procedure until he was able to initiate the actions on his own, and then raised the level of difficulty by asking him to perform the activity to the beat of a metronome. I then asked Teddy to point to numbers arranged in two vertical columns alternating in sequence from 1 to 10. (For more detail about these procedures, see Chapter 9.) Finally, I scattered numbers on the chalkboard and asked Teddy to point to them in sequence, an activity that required figure/ground discrimination and called on both ambient and focal visual function. Thanks to Teddy's obsession with numbers, he cooperated enthusiastically in these procedures.

The resulting flow of neural motor information led to an "awakening" that allowed Teddy, over time, to achieve a much higher level of visual performance. He went on to speak 75 words, and, within eight months, he was speaking in two- and three-word phrases. He developed an interest in sports, and could listen to and watch television at the same time.

Bobby: The teenager who talked to himself

Bobby, a 14-year-old with autism, was 6 feet tall and quite a handful. Constantly in motion, he talked to himself ceaselessly. His receptive language appeared intact, because he would respond well when asked to perform a task, but he would not converse with anyone. His visual attention was fleeting. My visual analysis showed that his eyes were free of pathology, and a matching task indicated 20/20 acuity without glasses.

On the Kaplan Nonverbal Battery, Bobby responded well to yoked base-up prisms when seated and watching the video, but his hyperactive behavior continued. He could stand and rock on the rocking board while watching the video, but he attended to the television only for brief periods, and he repeatedly stepped off the board and talked to himself. During the ball play task, the yoked base-up prisms had little effect: he continued talking and moving, and rather than catching the ball, he batted it away. This last behavior was an important clue indicating that Bobby had a visual timing problem.

Bobby's problems stemmed from developmental delays in spatial organization. A child or adult with such delays will compress the visual field to what can be controlled.

A visual field is composed of both figure and ground. Attention to the field is determined by perceptual style: a global style tends to pay attention to "ground," while a focal style tends to pay attention to "figure." Bobby had a global style, resulting in a "scan path" eye movement pattern—a fast alternating attention to ground that is an attempt to resolve the conflicts in the fields being viewed. He was "all ground and no figure," the opposite of what I see in patients with a focal style (one of whom I'll discuss later) who are "all figure and no ground."

Bobby's behaviors were an attempt to maintain his version of "normal"—the solution that allowed him to create some sense of balance with his world. He had severe spatial organization deficits because his global perceptual style caused a mismatch between where objects were and where they appeared to be. This forced him to make excessive eye movements to find what he was looking for, interfering with visual thinking and speech and affecting him emotionally. He also exhibited orientation problems, and his hyperactivity and hyperverbosity were logical adaptations, because both provided cues that allowed him to maintain a body schema. Again, however, this left him little energy for other motor and cognitive skills.

To help Bobby to create new and better solutions, I planned a visual management program that would increase his visual attention and slow him down. I also introduced him to the concept that attending to the environment could be pleasurable rather than painful.

We started with a ball-catching task. The act of catching a ball, a global task, requires selective attention to two aspects of the visual system: movement and depth. When visual attention is established, the hands will move reflexively. However, when movement and depth are not established, the mind leads and causes the body to avoid or defend against the ball, which is what occurred in Bobby's case.

By modifying the task of ball play, I allowed Bobby to succeed at the act of catching. Since he couldn't deal with "self" and space at the same time, I had him perform the task seated in order to reduce his need to attend to gravitational input (a challenge for patients with an impaired body schema). Second, I compensated for his impaired perception of form by substituting a 9-inch balloon for the smaller ball. This gave him a more global target, as well as more time to respond. Rather than asking Bobby to catch the balloon, I asked him to bunt it with a rolling pin. In time, he was able to switch from the balloon to a ball, and he could attend in a relaxed way and enjoy the activity. Improvements occurred in his inward and outward vergence, causing better depth perception and timing.

Initially, Bobby used excessive body movements when he walked. To change this behavior, we needed to generate a spatial rearrangement that would force Bobby to pay attention. To do this, I used disruptive yoked prisms, and had Bobby practice the "walk and sit" procedure outlined in Chapter 3. As a result, Bobby's hyperactivity diminished greatly.

Pleased by the success of the disruptive yoked prisms, I used them again in the next procedure. Sitting Bobby down, I placed 20-diopter prisms on him, base-up in front of the right eye and base-down in front of the left eye, with anaglyph red and green lenses. With the glasses in place, I asked Bobby to look at a 2½-inch ball positioned at chest level on a string. Holding the ball, I started to move it. Bobby's eyes followed, and I asked him, "How many balls do you see?" He answered, "Two." At this point, his mother, startled, told me, "He never answers questions." During this activity, Bobby also stopped talking to himself, and his mother reported that he refrained from this behavior until they returned home.

Bobby is still undergoing visual training, and is consolidating his gains. How much progress he will make remains to be seen, but so far, the results are highly encouraging and his family is very excited by his improvement.

Sean: Choosing what to see

Some of the most interesting research I've read in recent years was reported by Margaret Livingstone and David Hubel, whose work focuses on how we perceive art. Their research indicates that vision, depth, movement, color, and form perception are handled by entirely separate channels in the nervous system. In discussing visual perception, Livingstone and Hubel write:

> Anatomical and physiological observations in monkeys indicate that the primate visual system consists of several separate and inde-
> pendent subdivisions that analyze different aspects of the same

retinal image: cells in cortical visual areas 1 and 2 and higher visual areas are segregated into three interdigitating subdivisions that differ in their selectivity for color, stereopsis, movement, and orientation. The pathways selective for form and color seem to be derived mainly from the parvocellular geniculate subdivisions, the depth- and movement-selective components from the magnocellular. At lower levels, in the retina and in the geniculate, cells in these two subdivisions differ in their color selectivity, contrast sensitivity, temporal properties, and spatial resolution.[1]

These different subdivisions of vision became obvious to me when I found that I could relate the psychophysiological behaviors of individuals to the selectivity of their visual perception. For example, I once evaluated an art gallery owner who showed deficits in depth perception. When I asked him, "How do you choose your paintings—by color?" He replied, "Exactly." Another acquaintance, an artist who avoided landscapes and produced her work from her mind rather than what she viewed, had problems with the subdivisions of depth and movement.

Sean, a young patient of mine, was lower functioning than these individuals, but he too exhibited the effects of selectively shutting down visual channels. A high-functioning ten-year-old with Asperger Syndrome, Sean was highly articulate and talked constantly. He was hyperactive, was easily frightened by unexpected sights or sounds, and had problems with eye–hand coordination and social interaction. He attended a regular neighbourhood school and performed at grade level, but his reading was slow and his organization of space on a page appeared to be a problem. He displayed delays in both general and specific motor functioning.

Sean's performance on the modified Van Orden Star test offered more insight into his visual deficits. His lines were unorganized patterns projected below the spatial midline. His left apex was fan-shaped, and the right apex was open. The implication was that although his performance indicated a global perceptual style, he was overcompensated and behaving as a focal performer. He also was beginning to use his right eye for far vision, and his left eye for near vision. His convergence measurements showed high break and low recovery, revealing a tenacity of will and a lack of resilience. All in all, his results indicated a high expenditure of energy for small amounts of reward.

Sean was like a four-cylinder operating on two cylinders. He selected color and form, while suppressing depth and movement. In designing a treatment for Sean, I recognized that he had chosen to be a focal performer in order to maintain control of his environment and acheive homeostasis. Thus, I began with his strengths and moved gradually to his weaknesses, in order to limit his anxiety and prevent him from becoming overwhelmed. The initial stages of Sean's vision therapy program focused on gradually moving him from inside his visual tunnel to outside of the tunnel. When he was comfortable outside the tunnel, I switched to disruptive lenses in order to force him to open up blocked visual channels so that he could again see color and movement.

I see many patients who, like Sean, struggle to function at high levels even though they see only a partial picture of their world. Most of the time, they have no idea that there's something wrong with what they see. One six-year-old, for instance, had double vision. I demonstrated this by holding a pen light in front of one of his eyes, covering the other eye with a red lens, and then removing the cover from the first eye. I asked him what he saw, and he said, "A red light and a white light." "That's seeing double," I told him. "Doesn't everybody?" he asked.

While tuning out some channels makes the world less threatening to patients with visual deficits, it also degrades their performance. Good vision depends on our ability to correlate input from all of the visual subdivisions into a coherent whole, and the patient who cannot do this is missing crucial pieces of the puzzle. The more we can empower patients to open up these suppressed channels, the more proficient they will become.

Bernard: The effects of "frozen" vision

Bernard was nine years old when I first saw him. At that time, he exhibited delays in both general and specific motor skills, and his eyes or mouth appeared to "freeze" at times. He could read the New York Times, but he didn't understand what he was reading. Although he could hear when people talked to him, he had a timing problem and had trouble understanding what was said to him. The teachers at his special school had to constantly repeat their instructions in order for him to understand.

My evaluation showed that Bernard responded positively to yoked base-down prisms. The lenses improved his response to gravity, his balance, his gait, and his ability to catch a ball. I was optimistic about his prognosis, based on the changes I observed with the lenses.

Bernard's spatial organization was tunneled, and he was "all figure and no ground" (the opposite of Bobby, whose case I discussed earlier). He operated on color and form, while blocking out eye movement and depth perception. His behaviors—touching objects, moving to objects to inspect them rather than observing them from a distance—were typical of a person having trouble answering the question of "Where is it?" rather than "What is it?"

I placed Bernard in a visual management program in which he raised his level of performance in general and specific motor tasks. His spoken language went from short phrases to full sentences, and he developed a sense of humor. He still had problems in comprehending other people's speech, and his eye movements were still frozen. However, like many other children on the autism spectrum, he found a way to catch a ball, walk, and navigate his surroundings without too much difficulty.

Years later, when Bernard was 16, I received a call from his mother. She wanted to re-start his therapy, hoping that we could move his comprehension skills to a higher level.

My testing at this point revealed that during the ball play task, Bernard could see a ball swung across him at chest level in the frontal plane, but could not track it. As part of his new therapy program, I introduced the activity described earlier, placing disruptive prisms (one base-up and one base-down) and red/green anaglyphs over Bernard's eyes. As he tracked the ball, I asked him, "What do you see?" He immediately replied that he saw two balls, one red and one green. Within seconds, I noticed that his eyes were starting to move and his body language—lowered shoulders, looser facial expression—indicated a greater degree of relaxation. I followed this procedure with the "Lazy Eight" procedure described earlier, again using disruptive lenses. I then took out a reading chart and asked Bernard to read the first paragraph to me. He read fluently, and when I asked him to describe what he'd read, he was quite accurate. These simple procedures had moved Bernard to a higher level of comprehension, which was consolidated over time.

Bernard had chosen to constrain movement and depth in order to avoid double vision. As a result, he lost his ability to trust his space world. What my procedures accomplished, by taking away the ability of

Bernard's neuromuscular system to even attempt to fuse the images he saw, was what A.M. Skeffington called "breaking the space lattice"—an act that forced him to reconstruct his spatial world. The color cues heightened Bernard's trust in his perception: even though he was aware that only one ball existed, he could trust the illusion of two balls, leaving each eye free to move. This in turn freed the flow of energy and information to his higher cortical processes, completing the cycle of movement, information, and execution.

Bernard's case and others in this chapter highlight what I said earlier about vision being not a matter of passive perception, but rather an active process of intelligence. We take it for granted that what we see is a real picture of our surroundings, but in reality, it is largely a construct built by our brains. As Skeffington's classic "four circles" diagram (see Chapter 2, Figure 2.1) shows, what we see is the end result of the visual process combining multiple channels of information into a coherent whole.

Our goal, in therapy, is to facilitate this integration, thus giving our patients a more complete and accurate picture of their world and their place in it. The result, as one parent put it in describing the changes in her autistic daughter, is "a more vital, vibrant person"—someone who can spend each day exploring and enjoying the world, rather than trying to escape from it.

Note

1 Livingstone, M. and Hubel, D. (1988) "Segregation of form, color, movement, and depth: Anatomy, physiology, and perception." *Science 240*, 740–749.

CHAPTER 9

What Does Breathing Have to do with Vision?

As you read these words, you're probably breathing smoothly and easily, without even realizing that you're doing it. That's because breathing is largely a self-regulating process, controlled by the involuntary nervous system.

If I entered your room right now and held a gun to your head, however, your breathing would change dramatically. Breathing responds to any impact on the system, whether it is a threatening stranger, a frightening traffic incident, or the effort of walking down an icy, slippery street. We hold our breath under shock, and we sigh to restore our breath when we are experiencing acute stress. We also alter our breathing patterns in response to chronic stressors, whether emotional or physical, and these patterns can become ingrained and dysfunctional. Such dysfunctional breathing patterns are a very common problem in the patients I see, and they contribute significantly to visual dysfunction.

Breathing, like any other reflex activity, is genetically imbedded. However, all reflexes must learn to integrate with visual motor function in order to become optimal. This integration is affected by experience, and thus open to change. Because constraints on breathing affect every aspect of performance, an effective vision therapy program must incorporate remediation of the inappropriate breathing patterns that many patients have developed.

A high percentage of patients with developmental delays, and particularly those on the autism spectrum, exhibit dysfunctional breathing patterns stemming from delays in neuromotor development. Evidence of this problem can be seen in their low muscle tone, their postural warps, and their inability to blow out candles, blow bubbles, or play instruments such as whistles or flutes that require skill in breathing. Additional symptoms of breathing problems include yawning or sighing, which are efforts to exchange carbon dioxide for oxygen. It also is common to see patients with autism holding their breath when moving their eyes to locate objects, because they do not possess the efficient neuromotor synergies that would allow them to breathe and move their eyes at the same time.

One effect of dysfunctional breathing is a high level of tension and anxiety. Breathing expert Carola Speads notes, "The quality of our breathing determines the quality of our lives. Health, moods, energy, creativity—all depend on the oxygen supply provided by our breathing. But the pressures of our modern-day life have created an almost literally breathless culture." This is especially true for autistic children, whose high stress levels and inability to move and breathe, due to lack of synergistic action on the part of their neuromuscular complexes, have left them "breathless."

Normal breathing reduces tension, releasing energy and allowing us to pay attention to our surroundings. In patients with autism or related disorders, an inability to integrate the physiological functions of movement and breathing leads to overly tense muscles, reduces attention, and stresses the nervous system. This tension in turn impairs vision, leading to mismatches between where things are and where they appear to be, or in more severe cases, to a total immobility of the eye.

My clinical experience is that fear and anxieties are common in patients with global perceptual styles, and that the severity of these emotional problems often correlates with the level of breathing dysfunction. It is not uncommon to see hyperventilation in children with autism spectrum disorders or developmental delays, and this hyperventilation can lead to apnea and/or panic attacks. Some of the behaviors seen in children with autism spectrum disorders (e.g., breath-holding, inability to blow out candles) may indeed be learned responses that developed as an attempt to prevent hyperventilation and the resulting feelings of anxiety.

Reading is another action that is powerfully affected by disturbances in breathing. I've treated many children who hold their breath while reading, because they are physically unable to breathe and read at the same time. The result is reduced attention to the words on the page, a tense posture while reading, continual yawning and sighing to replenish depleted oxygen supplies, and a high level of stress.

Postural warps, too, can be a consequence of faulty breathing. Physiologist V.S. Gurfinkel noted that in normal breathing, the upper and middle parts of the torso subtly move backward during inhalation and forward during exhalation. At the same time, the hips make a move of equal size in the opposite direction. The purpose of these movements is to maintain the position of the head, in order to optimize visual and auditory perception. This synergy of torso and hip muscles does not occur in patients with autism or related disabilities; what we see, instead, is an oscillation of the center of gravity coinciding with the phase of respiration. This change in the body's center of gravity causes corresponding changes in posture, gait, and movement, and it contributes to toe-walking as well as the rigidity often seen in patients with autism. In addition, it can lead to functional scoliosis or lesser spinal curvatures.

In an earlier chapter, I described a teenager whose scoliosis improved from a 20-degree to a 12-degree curvature during the course of vision therapy, eliminating the need for surgery. Ronnie, a ten-year-old with scoliosis and learning problems, was another success story.

My evaluation of Ronnie showed a global perceptual style, delays in orientation, and inefficient breathing patterns including breath-holding. I prescribed directive yoked prisms for full-time wear and disruptive yoked prisms for spatial rearrangement, and implemented a therapy program designed to raise Ronnie's conscious awareness of kinesthetic and visual interaction. Breathing procedures played a prominent role in this treatment plan.

Ronnie responded beautifully to therapy, overcoming his learning disabilities and becoming a high-achieving student. Moreover, he now has no noticeable scoliosis.

Another characteristic of individuals with autism or developmental disabilities is a rocking motion, which compensates for the lack of synergistic neural control of the triad of eyes, head, and body. Here again, breathing impairments play a role. One of my patients, a five-year-old diagnosed with PDD, constantly rocked his head when he watched TV, walked, or ran. One month into a program incorporating movement and breathing procedures, his head-rocking had diminished so much that his parents continually commented on the stillness of his posture.

Such changes are evidence that vision therapy affects neuromotor organization and re-establishes new synergies, a union of several muscles (however distant from each other) into a single control group. One of these is a "respiratory synergy" of the vertical posture that must be addressed in order to improve performance.

Tony, a 16-year-old whose parents asked me to address his learning difficulties, exhibited a global style and was tightly organized. My evaluation indicated that he had an overcompensated global style and, as a result, tunneled his spatial world. He was also a shallow breather.

As I previously mentioned, I don't take patients' histories before I examine them. The information I gleaned from my evaluation of Tony was sufficient for me to predict his behaviors, performance, and symptoms, without questioning him or his parents.

In trying to gain Tony's confidence, I decided not to talk about academics, because this was not a comfortable topic for him. Instead, I asked him, "Do you play sports?"

He answered, "Yes."

"What sport?"

"Lacrosse."

"What position? Defense?"

He nodded. I asked him, "How bad are your lower back pains at the end of the game?"

He was taken aback, and said, "How do you know about my back pains? I never told anyone."

I knew then that I had his attention. I said, "Would it be helpful if I could improve your ability to see a greater part of the field, improve your timing, and get rid of your back pain?" He replied, "If you can do that, I would love to do vision training."

How did I know about Tony's back problems, and how did I know that vision training could alleviate them? As I've noted, the upper torso normally bends forward during exhalation. In Tony's case, he held his breath and locked his posture into a compressed forward position in order to reduce the field to what he could control. When a player or ball came within his "tunnel" he could react; however, it was difficult for him to be aware of movement occurring outside of this area. His natural athletic ability had carried him to the varsity level, but his tunnel vision and the backaches and fatigue caused by his abnormal breathing limited his ability to elevate his performance—as well as his ability to attend to academics.

I planned a visual management program for Tony that helped him develop movement and breathing synergies, as well as addressing his tunneled vision. As a result, Tony elevated his game, and his posture became more normal. He was thrilled at his enhanced sports performance, and his parents were even more pleased by his improved grades.

To understand the breathing problems common in children with autism or other developmental delays, it is useful to understand the normal embryological development of breathing behavior. Although a child takes its first breath of air only after birth, the process of breathing is well established in the womb, where this skill develops in four stages as outlined by Arnold Gesell:

- *Spasm:* Early in development, the fetus responds to a tap on the face by twitching its head and rotating toward the stimulus. Around the 38th day of fetal development, the diaphragm will twitch once or twice if the fetus is tapped on the face. This is the first use of a specific respiratory muscle.

- *Rhythm:* Around the 40th day of development, diaphragmatic spasms start to occur in a rhythmic pattern, eventually occurring more than 60 times per minute, and the intercostal muscles involved in respiration begin to function.

- *Segregation:* At this point, around the 45th day of development, the fetus will respond to a tap on the face by moving the entire body. The movements of the diaphragm and chest, however, will last longer than the movements of the other parts of the body. From this point on, the respiratory rhythm becomes more independent, more prominent, and more intense.

- *Inhibition:* At this stage, the fetus does not respond with a spasmodic movement if touched. However, if the fetal oxygen supply from the placental cord is reduced, the fetus will respond by reverting to the "segregation" stage of breathing, and then successively to the two previous stages. As Gesell noted, "This is a striking example of the hierarchy of controls which is characteristic of the embryology of behavior."[1]

Like the fetus, the child or adult with breathing difficulties due to poor muscle tone often reverts to earlier stages of development of the respiratory system. Normally, there is a structural organization of the nervous system's control of respiration, starting with the movement of the diaphragm and moving to movement of the neck and torso muscles. When this sequence cannot occur smoothly and rhythmically, due to maturational delays and a patient's adaptive responses, an enormous amount of effort and energy must be devoted simply to breathing. All other performance is impaired when breathing is impaired, because breathing sustains and regulates the activities of the central nervous system.

As I've noted, the parents of my patients often exhibit milder versions of their children's problems. A case in point involved Jack, a 45-year-old man who brought his son to be treated for visual problems causing learning disabilities.

When I met with Jack, it became obvious that he too had significant visual and breathing problems. In college, he'd played basketball because of his size—6 feet, 6 inches—but he was never a good shooter. Now, as an adult, he found his job so demanding that he slept half the day on Saturdays and Sundays just to have enough energy to face another week. His posture and gait were so awkward that at the age of 43 he'd needed two hip replacements.

My visual analysis showed that Jack had intermittent double vision, coupled with an inability to move his eyes and breathe at the same time. A visual management program, incorporating lenses and vision therapy and including breathing procedures, allowed him to become aware of his breathing and visual disorders and to overcome them.

In a short time, Jack found that he had far more energy and could enjoy his weekends instead of sleeping through them. He reported that movement was no longer a conscious experience of pain, but rather was a natural, automatic, and pleasurable act. This is the "aha" feeling that so often occurs when therapy allows a patient to experience the natural sense of well-being that comes from being able to move and breathe without constraint.

Fortunately, patients with inefficient breathing habits can unlearn these habits. With help, many individuals can learn to breathe in a relaxed and efficient way, and to coordinate their breathing easily with their movements. This results in better attention and mood, reduced anxiety and fearfulness, and a higher level of visual performance.

My own introduction to breathing and visual management came when I met the late Carola Speads, one of the world's leading teachers of relaxed, efficient breathing. When I arrived at her office, she greeted me and immediately asked me to take off my shoes and shirt. I thought this was strange, but she ushered me into a room where there were others in the same manner of dress. Carola directed us to sit on a low bench, and led us through a series of movements and breathing activities. As I followed her instructions, I began to sense that my eyes were relaxing, and that I could see more and more of the space surrounding me. Using her techniques in my own practice, I find that they can create this same sense of relaxation and expanded vision in both non-disabled and disabled patients, although some modifications are needed with the latter group.

A second person whose work influenced my understanding of the role of breathing in visual management was the late Moshe Feldenkrais, whose techniques are designed to raise performance by increasing self-awareness through movement. The Feldenkrais Method, taught world-wide, consists of movement sequences that create improved awareness of body parts or functions that were previously "neglected" or inefficiently used. Procedures include teaching students to become aware of, and have control over, voluntary aspects of breathing. "The advantage of a habit acquired by awareness," Feldenkrais said, "is that when it shows unfitness or maladjustment when confronted with reality, it easily provokes new awareness and so helps one to make a fresh and more efficient change."

I was also greatly influenced by the work of F.M. Alexander, whose Alexander Technique—developed in the early 1900s—is still in wide use a century later. Alexander's story is interesting: he began his career as a public speaker, but became so hoarse during recitals that he would lose his voice and gasp for air. Resting his voice helped, but the problem returned each time he went back to public speaking. Realizing that he must be doing something wrong, Alexander set out to discover what the problem was, observing himself carefully in the mirror while speaking normally and then while reciting in the manner he used for public speaking. He discovered that while speaking in his "elocutionist" voice, he pulled his head back, depressed his larynx, and sucked in his breath—a pattern that also occurred to a lesser degree during normal speaking. After several unsuccessful efforts to change this habit, he hit upon the approach of actively inhibiting his initial desire to speak, and giving himself directions to hold his head forward and up, with his back straight. This technique, which he termed "inhibition," became the foundation for the Alexander Technique, which begins by creating consciousness of inefficient breathing techniques so that they can be changed. In *The Lost Sixth Sense*, physiologist David Garlick describes Alexander's pioneering concept:

> Alexander ... showed a shrewd understanding of how the brain worked. Our consciousness, in the cortex of the brain, is where our will to do something arises. After this the pathways go to centres deep in the brain which form the subconscious or unconscious. If nothing is done to stop existing programs being activated resulting in inappropriate muscle contractions, then a person's characteristic way of sitting, standing and doing things will occur... Alexander made the significant discovery that the way to interrupt the sequence was to "will to do" something then stop (or inhibit) it which will allow a new "program" to be developed subsconsciously while consciously or mentally giving directions.[2]

I have combined the techniques and philosophies of Speads, Feldenkrais, and Alexander to create learning experiences that allow my patients to become aware of, and overcome, the breathing difficulties that interfere with their visual processes. The first step in helping patients learn to breathe efficiently is to introduce breathing skills in isolation. The next step is to integrate breathing with movement, so a smooth synergy is created.

Here are a few simple but highly effective techniques I recommend for accomplishing these goals:

- *Tissue breathing:* Have your patient lie on the floor, face up, while you hold the patient's hands to keep them immobile. Place a thin tissue over the patient's mouth and nose, to interfere with the normal intake of air. This forces the patient to remove the tissue by exhaling. In some cases, you may need to lend assistance by pressing gently on the patient's diaphragm. In time, the patient will succeed in learning how to exhale efficiently.

- *Bubble-blowing:* Demonstrate this activity, and then have the patient practice until the activity can be performed easily. It takes time and patience, but most children are fascinated with bubbles and will persevere in spite of the difficulty of the task. Similar activities include having children blow whistles or horns, or having them blow in a straw in a glass of water to make bubbles.

- *Straw paper or ping-pong ball blowing:* This is another excellent activity to use with nonverbal children. Seat your patient across from you at a table. Take the paper off a straw, roll the paper into a small ball, and blow it across the table, keeping an eye on your patient's reaction. At first, the child will reach out and manipulate the paper, indicating a motivation to imitate the task. When this occurs, take the paper ball and place it front of your patient. More often than not, the patient will try to initiate the action you performed. When this happens, two things are accomplished: the patient becomes aware of the physiological process of breathing, and the patient tracks the movement with his or her eyes in the sagittal plane.

  To make this procedure even easier, you can use a ping-pong ball rather than the paper. The ball rolls easily, requiring less force of exhalation and reducing the volume of breath needed. Using red and green anaglyph lenses will provide color cues and stimulate binocular awareness.

- *Dowel procedures:* The seated and standing dowel procedures described in Chapter 7 are highly effective in creating movement and breathing synergies, resulting in a marked relaxation response and a much better ability to attend to the environment.

The dowel activities outlined in Chapter 7, and used so successfully with Rachelle (see below), address movement and respiration. In the next procedure I describe, we increase the level of complexity by asking the patient to add eye movement. This aids patients in creating the synergies needed to successfully combine breathing, moving, and seeing.

Rachelle, a 35-year-old patient, was referred by her psychiatrist because of the role vision was playing in her anxiety and depression. After she spent six months in therapy with me, her psychiatrist was able to reduce her medication. She returned to work, and once again began enjoying social interaction.

One year later, during a very hot spell in May, Rachelle was in a car accident that affected her speech, posture, and attention. Her husband called me to tell me about the accident and to say that Rachelle had stopped communicating and appeared completely "out of it."

I told him to bring her to my office. She arrived wearing a winter coat, gloves, and a wool hat. Her head was cocked to one side, and her husband had to support her as she walked. My first thought was that if I could stimulate a synergy of breathing and movement, it might help her to relax and attend.

I sat Rachelle down and placed a dowel in her hands. With my hands inside hers, I began moving the dowel up and down, pausing in the middle. In time, I felt Rachelle relax. Slowly, she started to participate in the movement. I then started moving the dowel to the right and back to center, and then left and back to the center. As I continued over a period of two or three minutes, I could feel her movements begin to flow.

I asked Rachelle to breathe, exaggerating my own exhalations as a guide. In a short period, a most exciting event occurred. Rachelle stopped the activity, straightened her posture, and reached up, taking off her hat. Her first words were, "It's awfully hot in here." She proceeded to take off her gloves and coat. By the time the session ended, Rachelle was quite articulate, and she was able to walk out without assistance.

Dowel, arrow, and breathe

The procedure requires a chalkboard and the same dowel used in the previous procedures. Later steps require a rocking board.

Procedure

Begin with the patient standing, in order to assess how well earlier neural synergies have been established. If the patient has problems at any point, proceed with the patient seated in order to ensure success and maximize motivation.

On a chalkboard, write the numbers 1 and 2 on the same level, 18 inches apart, and draw a line between them. Ask the patient to put his or her finger on number 1 and trace the line to number 2. Next, ask the patient to move his or her finger across the line, breathing on the finger as if "blowing" it across the line. Then ask the patient to hold a dowel in both hands, with the hands separated a distance slightly wider than the body. The patient should move the dowel to the left of the body in line with number 1, while inhaling. Then the patient should move the dowel to the right of the body, in line with the number 2, while simultaneously exhaling, stopping when the dowel and the eyes reach the 2. After a brief relaxation, the patient should repeat this process.

This is followed by arranging numbers in two columns:

1	2
3	4
5	6
7	8
9	10

The patient now exhales while moving the dowel from odd to even numbers, and inhales while moving from even to odd. You will notice that the patient is making a "Z" pattern, similar to the pattern in which the eyes move during reading. Initially, lines should be used to mark the correct path. When the child is proficient, the lines should be removed. The procedure is repeated with the patient standing on a rocking board.

As a new synergy of action is established during this procedure, you will see your patient become more confident in moving, seeing, and breathing. Eye tracking will progress from a fixational focal ability to saccadic global ability, and figure/ground perception will begin to be established. These changes will liberate energy previously needed to process seeing, moving, and breathing in isolation. The resulting orchestration of the sensory input often leads to increased verbalization, with nonverbal patients frequently exhibiting echolalia at this stage.

The dowel procedures I've described are designed to introduce new synergies of movement and breathing. The next stage is to show patients how these new skills can facilitate their interaction with their space-world. Following dowel training, I have patients blow and then bunt a balloon, and then blow at it and bunt it simultaneously. Anaglyph lenses are added to provided additional depth and movement cues.

When I work with verbal adults, they often tell me that performing these breathing, movement and attention tasks initiates a relaxation response. Children who are nonverbal or unable to express their feelings will reveal this change in their body language, by moving more fluidly and progressing from tapping the balloon with the rolling pin to smashing it vigorously while smiling or laughing.

Other activities that are effective at this stage include breathing activities with anaglyphs, viewing a white paper while rocking on the balance board, or walking on a 2-by-4 rail. These interactions of kinesthetic and visual modalities, when mastered, will reach automaticity.

With high-functioning patients, I like to use a two-part breathing procedure that is an expansion of an activity used by Carola Speads. I have revised her procedure slightly because the original version requires time and patience, while mine offers immediate gratification—an important factor in keeping patients motivated. Here are the two steps of the activity.

Straw procedure

Part I

Have your patient sit in an erect position, holding one end of a straw between the lips and holding the other end of the straw between the thumb and index finger as if holding a pencil. Ask the patient, "When you look at your fingers, how many straws do you see?" If the patient replies, "One," he or she is suppressing an eye. If the patient sees two straws, he or she is using both eyes.

Next, ask, "Do the two straws appear to make a 'V' or an 'X' or two parallel lines?" The correct answer is a "V." If the straws appear to make an X or parallel lines, there is a mismatch between where the patient is aiming his or her eyes and where the fingers are in space. The X is overconvergence, and the parallel lines are underconvergence.

Have your patient move his or her fingers back and forth along the straw, from the mouth to the other end of the straw. As the fingers move away from the mouth, the straw should begin to appear as an X in the middle of the straw, and then appear as a "V" when the fingers reach the end. As the fingers near the lips, this process should reverse (see illustration below).

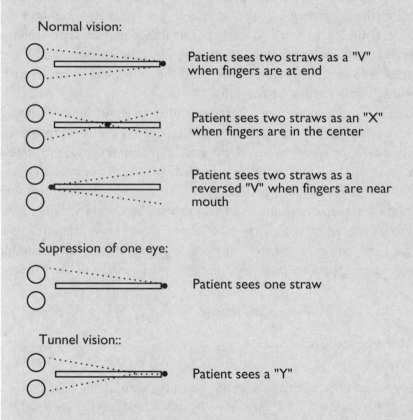

Normal vision:

Patient sees two straws as a "V" when fingers are at end

Patient sees two straws as an "X" when fingers are in the center

Patient sees two straws as a reversed "V" when fingers are near mouth

Supression of one eye:

Patient sees one straw

Tunnel vision::

Patient sees a "Y"

If your patient suppresses an eye or exhibits a mismatch, add another visual cue by having the patient wear red/green lenses. In some cases, this breaks the suppression. If the patient sees an X, have him or her look at a point in space beyond the fingers, or place a pencil beyond the fingers and have the patient look at the pencil. Move the pencil farther out, until the straws become a "V." This gives the patient feedback about the mismatch. If the patient sees parallel lines, hold the pencil in front of the patient's fingers.

Part II

Ask your patient to breathe through the straw, while holding it in the same manner as in Part I. Encourage the patient to become aware of his/her abdominal and trunk muscles and overall muscle tone. This will reduce tension, while increasing the flow of air.

As in Part I, have your patient move his or her fingers back and forth along the straw, from the mouth to the other end of the straw. When the patient's fingers move toward the mouth, the patient should breathe out, and when they move toward the other end of the straw, he or she should inhale. The optimal visual respiratory synergy occurs when your patient is able to breathe comfortably and obtain the proper perceptual information from the straw. It is advantageous to have your patient hold his or her free hand close to the straw opening before and after practicing, to confirm that the breath coming out of the straw is warm, a sign of deep rather than superficial breathing.

One of my patients, a young woman named Nora, worked as a cashier in a department store. On one very busy Saturday, a large number of shoppers crowded around Nora's station. Conscious of their impatience, Nora tried to speed up to accommodate them. Looking up at the customers, and then down at the cash register, she suddenly became dizzy and blacked out.

Alarmed by the incident, Nora went to her internist, who referred her to me. Her visual findings on the Keystone Skills, Van Orden Star, and the 21-point battery indicated a highly disorganized global perceptual style. Her symptoms were similar to pseudo-coriolis, a syndrome involving vertigo and dizziness. (A real coriolis effect is caused by a structural disorder of the ear, while a pseudo-coriolis effect stems from eye movement disturbances affecting the neural labyrinth.)

When asked to walk to a mirror and then walk backward, Nora became highly stressed and nearly fainted. I asked her to repeat the task wearing plano yoked 2-diopter base-up prisms. This time she was much more in control, and walked forward and back with no difficulty.

I used Carola Speads' straw technique to check Nora's breathing capacity. First, I asked Nora to hold the straw in her mouth and place her free hand over the other opening of the straw. I then asked her to blow through the straw, feel the air coming out the other end, and tell me if it was warm or cold. She replied, "Cold," telling me that she was a shallow breather.

I prescribed yoked prisms and initiated a visual management program incorporating movement, breathing, and vision procedures. Nora recovered, and never had another attack.

While Nora was in training, her internist referred her to a cardiologist. His tests revealed a mitral valve prolapse—that is, a heart valve flap closing out of rhythm, causing a loss of blood flow. The cardiologist told Nora that her dizziness and fainting had been induced by stress, which can greatly increase the intensity or frequency of symptoms associated with mitral valve prolapse. Given the effectiveness of breathing therapy for Nora, I speculate that her abnormal breathing caused both her pseudo-coriolis symptoms and the exacerbation of her mitral valve prolapse, possibly through mechanisms involving excess stimulation of the vagal nerve.

When patients master breathing procedures and develop optimal respiratory synergies, you will frequently see marked improvements in posture, gait, and general mood and relaxation. In addition, improvements in reading and other academic work are often substantial.

Ari, a 16-year-old high school junior, had a history of multiple operations for strabismus (esotropia) at the age of three. Ari's doctors told his parents at the time of the surgeries that Ari's eyes would be cosmetically straight but would never work together, and that he would sometimes experience diplopia. Ari arrived at my office with a label of learning disability and a poor self-image in spite of years of psychological therapy. His low self-esteem wasn't surprising, because he was very clumsy and performed poorly in both academics and sports.

Ari responded to base-down and base-right yoked prisms, and within six months of training he exhibited flat fusion, improved posture, and a happier mood. The activities I'd recommended were successful, but not completely so: Ari could perform, but he could not sustain or establish depth, and his eyes always hurt.

At this time, I was just beginning to use breathing activities in my practice on a regular basis. I asked Ari to perform the straw activity described earlier in this chapter, and as he complied, he grabbed his eyes in pain. I never determined whether this was real physical pain, or a defense Ari used to avoid the task. In either case, it was temporary, and within two weeks Ari could perform the procedure easily and painlessly.

I decided to provide Ari with concrete evidence of the change that had occurred in his perception as a result of the straw activity. Using two identical vectograms, one placed at ortho and the other placed at "6" in a base-out position, I asked, "When you look at the top picture, is the clown single—and when you look at the bottom, is the quoit single?" He answered "yes" to both questions. Next, I told him, "When you look at the clown, relax, and when you look at the quoit, breathe out in a steady stream. Now, tell me what you see." Ari responded, "The quoit is floating off the screen." This, of course, was exactly the right answer. After a year of training, Ari had made his breakthrough and could perceive depth—an ability that greatly enhanced his performance in the classroom and on the playing field. He went on to graduate from college and, last I heard, is a highly successful businessman.

In a number of cases, breathing problems can be remedied by addressing other postural or behavioral issues. For example, children with autism or developmental delays often will tighten their facial muscles in an attempt to isolate eye muscle control. This leads to tooth-grinding, or to an exaggerated movement of the jaw. I often ask verbal children who are seated and tracking a ball moving side-to-side, "Does your jaw feel tight or loose?" Almost universally, those with breathing and spatial organization disorders will respond that it feels tight. The application of yoked base-up prisms often will cause the jaw to relax during tracking. In the case of patients with both orientation and organization problems, the addition of a beanbag placed on the head will aid in eliciting jaw relaxation. This relaxation of facial muscles leads in turn to an increased flow of oxygen, and a return to a rhythmic breathing.

Patience is key to success

The changes brought about by improved breathing are exciting and gratifying. However, it's important to realize, in working with patients with autism or other developmental delays, that you cannot "make" them breathe correctly. You can only encourage them to experiment with changing their breathing patterns on their own. Begin by analyzing their current breathing patterns, and then provide the tools most likely to help them change these patterns—bubbles, dowel movements, etc.—and let their responses develop as freely as possible.

As you experiment with different stimuli, your patients will eventually develop a harmony of visual-motor activity, releasing the breathing reflex to reach its full maturation. Autistic patients in particular need a good deal of time to become aware of their breathing reactions, and then must go through a stage of paying attention to their breathing before reaching a stage of automacity. Be patient, and let them set the pace.

With time, your patients will develop new synergies that will make the breathing process more automatic and natural. These changes are not conscious, but you will observe them in your patients' performance in the form of better posture, less toe-walking, greater relaxation, better attention to tasks, happier mood, better reading ability, and improved behavior. As patients consciously experience the natural rhythm of normal breathing, they will experience great satisfaction and a sense of physical well-being and calmness.

Because breathing patterns are unique to each individual, there is no cookbook approach to selecting breathing procedures. I strongly encourage visual management practitioners to investigate the works of Speads, Feldenkrais, and Alexander for additional insight into the types of breathing problems you are likely to encounter, and the most effective methods for addressing them. Breathing problems differ considerably from patient to patient, and while the simple procedures outlined in this chapter are a good start, you will find it necessary to tailor breathing activities individually for each patient, and sometimes to create your own.

Notes

1   Gesell, A. (1971) *The Embryology of Behavior: The Beginnings of the Human Mind.* Westport, CT: Greenwood Press.

2   Garlick, D. (1990) *The Lost Sixth Sense: A Medical Scientist Looks at the Alexander Technique.* Kensington, Australia: University of New South Wales. The history of Alexander's own vocal problems is related by Carol Porter McCullough (1996) in "The life and discovery of F.M. Alexander." In *The Alexander Technique and the String Pedagogy of Paul Rolland* (self-published).

CHAPTER 10

The Big Picture: Integrating Vision Therapy into a Comprehensive Treatment Program

My patients typically make remarkable progress, but I'm always careful to promise them or their families only what I can trust myself to deliver. Often, that is a great deal: improved speech, a happier mood, greater physical competence, less anxiety, better academic performance, and enhanced social skills. Other times, the improvements we see are limited by patients' resilience and motivation, or the degree of their neurological impairments.

In either case, I'm always aware that I am only one member of a team of specialists who will be helping my patient. Vision therapy is a powerful treatment, but it's only one of many therapies that autistic and other learning- and behavior-disordered individuals need. To achieve maximum benefit, vision therapy must be incorporated into a comprehensive treatment plan including educational, biochemical, and sensory integration approaches, and as vision professionals we need to understand and respect these other therapies.

This is particularly true in respect to children diagnosed with autism spectrum disorders. It is critical to address these disorders quickly, aggressively, and on many fronts simultaneously. Parents of autistic children typically are highly motivated and well-informed about current treatments, and clinicians should encourage and assist in their efforts to integrate vision therapy into an overall treatment "package" including the following approaches:

Applied Behavior Analysis

A key element of any autism treatment program is intensive educational intervention based on Applied Behavior Analysis (ABA). As I've noted, educational approaches cannot correct the underlying neurological deficits of autistic children in the ways that medical approaches can. However, early intervention using ABA (which is based on principles of behavior modification) is highly effective in helping children with autism spectrum disorders compensate for their disabilities, allowing many to make extraordinary progress. The majority of children who receive early ABA-based intervention acquire speech, and a high percentage—as many as half—achieve a level of performance that is normal or nearly normal.

Experts recommend that children with symptoms of autism begin receiving educational intervention immediately after diagnosis—typically between the ages of three and six—and even children under the age of two often respond dramatically. Vision professionals should be highly supportive of families' ABA programs, and should recommend such programs for any patients who are not already participating in them. For additional information on ABA, clinicians are referred to the works of Ivar Lovaas, Ph.D., who pioneered ABA treatment for children with autism.

Biomedical treatments

An equally important facet of an autism treatment program is biomedical intervention. This field is developing rapidly, with the former concept of autism as hopeless and incurable becoming outdated as doctors report remarkable progress or even outright cures in many cases. My colleague Bernard Rimland, Ph.D., a leader in this field, has founded the Defeat Autism Now! (DAN!) Project to promote research into the most promising biomedical treatments. Interested clinicians will find a wealth of information on biomedical approaches to autism treatment at his website, www.AutismResearchInstitute.com, or the website of my colleague Stephen M. Edelson, www.autism.org.

Clinicians whose patients' families are trying biomedical approaches should be aware that these treatments—while many are considered unproven by mainstream medicine—are proving to be highly beneficial for a large number of autistic children. Doctors using these techniques are in much the same position as visual management specialists, who encounter an enormous amount of skepticism even in the face of statistics showing that vision therapy works. Mounting evidence indicates that approaches such as gluten- and casein-free diets and other nutritional therapies can dramatically improve the behavior, communication, and cognitive performance of a significant percentage of children or adults with autism. Thus, it is vital for clinicians to keep an open mind about the biomedical approaches being used by parents of their patients, and to be supportive of these efforts.

Sensory therapies

Other approaches that benefit a number of autistic children include sensory integration therapy and auditory integration training (which can reduce hypersensitivity to sound, a common symptom in autism). Like vision therapy, these approaches enable children or adults with autism to reorganize their neural processes, often leading to permanent improvements in skills and behavior. If a parent is pursuing these therapies, you may wish to contact the practitioners providing them so that you can ensure that your efforts are well-coordinated.

Typically, parents report that all of these treatments—vision therapy, ABA, biomedical approaches, and other sensory approaches—have a synergistic effect. By supporting parents' efforts to pursue several or all of these avenues, and offering to coordinate efforts with other clinicians or educators, the visual management expert can greatly aid families in their quest to help their disabled children.

This quest, as dedicated clinicians soon learn, is an incredibly challenging one, but it is well worth the efforts of both parents and clinicians. As Steve Edelson notes, "The majority of autistic children can make enormous gains, and many can recover. The battle is long, hard, and often expensive, but it is a battle that can be won—and it is being won, by thousands of parents around the world." The same is true for patients with other developmental disabilities, learning disabilities, or mental illnesses. Thousands of these individuals, once consigned to failure or even institutionalization, are achieving levels of performance once believed to be impossible.

The visual management expert can play a key role in these victories, by correcting the debilitating visual deficits that would otherwise bar so many individuals with autism and related problems from reaching their full potential in life. I can guarantee, based on my own clinical experience, that there is no more challenging or rewarding task that the vision care professional can undertake—and no other patient population so desperately in need of our help.

The effects of vision therapy—in the words of patients, families, and doctors

I hope that the cases I've described in this book will inspire many of my colleagues to consider the field of developmental optometry. To offer additional insight into the rewarding nature of this profession, I would like to close this book with a selection of letters written by two parents, a patient, and one of my (once skeptical) colleagues:

> Such a wonderful change for my girl! In one year I have watched Leah go from a great avoidance of eye contact (when she did look at me, it was through a haze) to non-stop, right-at-me, wonderful eye contact (smiling eyes). She has gone from using the corners and tops of her eyes to focus on objects, to focusing with her head straight and eyes straight ahead. She used to wear sunglasses most of the time, as bright lights or sunlight would cause her to have seizures; now she wears them only occasionally, and not for very long. She used to hold on to railings with both hands while feeling with the bottoms of her feet in order to go up and down stairs; now she goes up and down without holding the rail. Before, she walked hunched over, while on her toes, and needed assistance most of the time, especially with stairs, curbs, or in a crowd. Now, she walks with a more confident, straight posture. NO MORE TOE WALKING! Before therapy, she was extremely stressed in crowds; now she enjoys including company in her favorite activities and will even sit at a table in a restaurant and socialize. She used to look down instead of at her surroundings; now she is very aware of the world and vocal about what she sees. Before, she would 'fold into herself' when hearing certain sounds; now she looks, and is not frightened.
>
> Leah is way more aware of what the kids her age and older are doing and likes to join in at age-level activities. She almost always has a smile on her face and is trying everything in her power to communicate. I can see a big improvement in her confidence, by the way she holds herself and looks us straight

in the eyes. Her attention span has also improved. Teachers, friends, and family have all commented on how Leah has "come out of her shell," and on her balance, eye contact, and soft, friendly smiles.

* * *

Jonathan has become a totally different person with a significantly higher level of confidence, which he couples with a new level of enthusiasm towards school, reading, and group sports activities. He is as aware as we are of the progress he has made, and he too credits this to both of your efforts... I credit you with giving him a totally new outlook on life, which he is beginning to see through his rose-colored glasses.

* * *

I came to you at age 47 not even realizing that I had a problem that could be solved. I just hit my 48th birthday and I want you to know what you have done for me. I was just out walking with my wife and, for the first time in my life, I saw the three-dimensional beauty of the area. The hills and the tree tops go all the way back to the sky. The empty areas between the leaves of trees are now filled with space. The beauty is incredible. However, if that was all you could do for me I would have felt unsatisfied.

As you know it used to take me five minutes to read a page, which I described as my biggest concern. Since the new reading glasses, combined with your training, I have now been able to double my reading speed on technical work and triple it on lighter reading. The first time you put prisms on me was the first time I realized what a headache was, because it went away. It was a shock to me to understand that everyone didn't see the way I did, and that my inability to see an entire face, because I had to focus so strongly on a particular piece such as an eye or a nose, was not the norm.

Your training has allowed me to drink in the broader views that I had to shut out before, while retaining my ability to concentrate... This has made me much calmer, more competent and confident with my clients...

I thank you from the bottom of my heart. My life is fuller and richer than I ever imagined thanks to what I have accomplished.

* * *

I have been treating schizophrenic and mental patients for four years now with the expected results. However, I must express my thanks to you personally, for the significant added improvement many of my patients have had once treated with yoked prisms and/or visual training.

Many excited expressions of thanks have come to me by satisfied (and honestly, very surprised) patients. Many feel for the first time they have a handle on their mental functioning. Just this morning I saw W— for his scheduled follow-up. He has struggled with troublesome hallucinations for years. Immediately after beginning to wear his prisms, his hallucinations became infrequent and subsequently stopped totally. He now remains five months without any hallucinations, thus allowing his [medication] dosage to be successfully lowered by significant amounts. Thank you for your part in the success of my patients.

As I share these and other success stories of my patients, I hope that I will inspire many readers to consider specializing in developmental optometry. Currently, optometry as a profession is expanding, but in the wrong direction—by trying to compete with ophthalmology for the 4 percent of patients with "hardware" problems such as refractive errors and cataracts. This is misguided, because millions of patients with "software" problems desperately need our help as well. As generalists, we can help not only people with overt ocular pathology, but also the huge numbers of people suffering with hidden visual problems that make their lives a constant struggle to survive. There is nothing more rewarding than seeing a patient speak for the first time, master a previously impossible academic skill, succeed at sports, or become less fearful and anxious, all as a result of vision therapy. This is why I still look forward to each day in the office, after more than four decades of practice—and why I highly recommend the field of developmental optometry for professionals who want their work to make a real difference to the world. With the numbers of individuals with autism, learning disabilities, and mental disorders burgeoning, there is tremendous need for practitioners in this field—and a tremendous opportunity to change your patients' lives for the better.

The Van Orden Star:
A Window Into Personal Space

The analysis of spatial behavior is, fundamentally, a description of the way behavior is conditioned by internal and external constraints. Skews of spatial orientation are brought about by visual adaptation to these two constraints. The Van Orden Star[1] probes the way we perceive, and mentally represent, the world around us. The Star can give insight into how we put this knowledge to work, and into action. In everyday life, we see coping patterns people have adopted in response to what they see and feel. There may be a turned foot, or a curved back; there may be heightened or lessened attention to a task. Coping patterns sometimes generate labels: dyslexic, autistic, emotionally disturbed, brain injured. Perceptual far- or near-point activities involve different levels of constraints. How an individual responds to these constraints is manifested in the way he modifies his drawing of the Van Orden Star patterns.

Weighting the scales in the search for balance

Harvard physiologist Walter B. Cannon proposed that all humans seek a position of homeostasis with their environment, a "steady state." Our bodies operate on a system of coordinates and axes of rotation (see Figure A.1).

When a body displays postural skews, it is responding to a misreading of spatial cues by the visual vergence system. Suppose we visualize the Van Orden Star pattern as an extension of the patient's perception of axes and planes in external space, as illustrated in Figure A.2. If the patient's Star drawing shows apices above or below primary gaze, or the target midline, he has demonstrated errors in vergence (see Figure A.3).

Execution of this pattern, while straightforward and simple, requires the individual to rapidly and accurately interpret what he sees, generate motor response, and maintain attention throughout. The appearance of his star pattern is, fundamentally, a predictor of the patient's spatial behavior. It reveals the way he responds to internal and external constraints. It depicts his particular version of homeostasis.

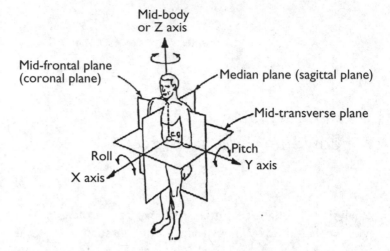

Figure A.1: Human system of coordinates and axes of rotation

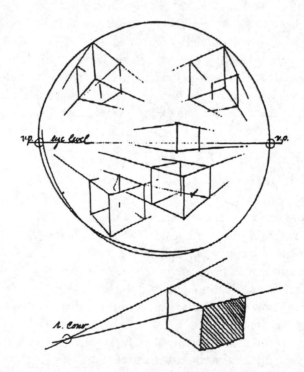

Figure A.2: Patient's perception of axes and planes in external space

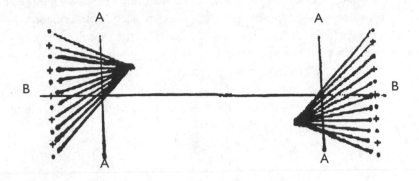

Figure A.3: Patient's errors in vergence

Instrumentation of the Van Orden Star

The keys to using any test are:

1. Understanding the demands of the test.

2. Keeping instructions consistent.

3. Making sure the available facts fit the model of interpretation.

The instrument of choice is the Correct-Eye-Scope with the transilluminated back. The Scope has an adjustable shaft with a Brewster stereoscope attached. The shaft marks dictate the visual distance to which the subject will attend. The standard design of the target, as designed by Van Orden, is a white translucent paper with two columns of figures, such as a star and a cross. Columns are composed of eleven figures placed 140 mm apart, for far-point testing (see Figure A.4).

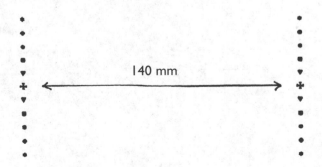

Figure A.4: Standard design for far-point testing

I use the standard Van Orden Star pattern, but in addition created a modification for near, so I might see the patient's response to near-point demands. If the distance star pattern represents a conflict between the visual and kinesthetic senses, but near-point activity usually creates the greatest stress, the adaptive response illustrated by the patient's star pattern would most likely be exacerbated at near. The second segment of testing is easily accomplished by adjusting the shaft to the near-point setting. A new test sheet is given, with the same columns of figures now 95 mm apart (see Figure A.5).

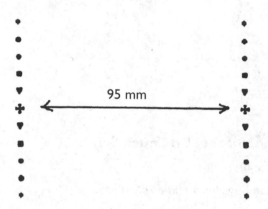

Figure A.5: Standard design for near-point testing

Figure A.6 is the star pattern of a six-year-old boy with learning-to-read difficulties. The distance star pattern was relatively as expected. The near pattern, however, displayed disorganization indicative of vergence dysfunction—a symptom, as we know, of reading difficulty.

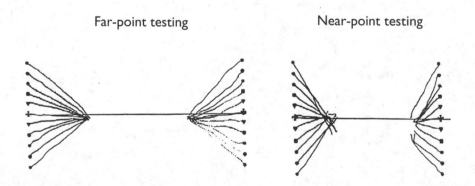

Figure A.6: Star pattern of a six-year-old boy with learning-to-read difficulties

Instructions to the patient

Direct the patient to please sit in front of the instrument and look through the eyepiece. Ask him or her "How many columns of figures do you see?" If the answer is two, ask, "Can you see both columns at the same time, or do they appear one at a time?" If the answer is the former, direct the patient to take two same-size pencils, one in each hand. Guide the patient to hold the pencils so as to write with them simultaneously. Ask him or her to place a pencil point on the center cross of each column—right pencil on the right cross, left on the left. Now ask, "Can you see both pencil points at the same time?" If yes, have him or her draw simultaneous lines, one toward the other, until the pencil points look as if they're touching. Next, place the left pencil on the top figure of the left column, and the right pencil on the bottom figure of the right. As before, the two pencils are to be brought toward each other until they appear to touch. The procedure is repeated with successive figures until the star pattern is complete.

Different patterns—different interpretations

In the optometric literature, several eminent authors have offered interpretations of the Van Orden Star, including Macdonald,[2] Quick,[3] Byall,[4] and, of course, Van Orden. All recognized some frequently seen pattern variations. Van Orden recognized the value of the Star for illustrating the balance between central and peripheral visual function. Macdonald's model has had the greatest influence on my thinking. He divided patients' patterns into four major classifications:

1. The tight peripheral-central relationship

2. The loosely organized peripheral-central relationship

3. A mismatch between peripheral visual and central visual function

4. A visual kinesthetic mismatch.

MacDonald as well as Van Orden both adhere to the model that an individual's perception of space influences his sensory system, and thus would influence that individual's drawing of the Star. A model is never right or wrong; it is based on the facts available at the time. Building on clinical experience, I was able to expand the model beyond the central-peripheral concept to include temporal and spatial factors as well.

The human organism is, after all, a spatial action system. Other organisms may depend more on other sensory modes, but in man, the visual sense dominates our sensory intake.

Human behavior is molded and conditioned by temporal and environmental constraints; these, in turn, affect all aspects of human performance. We seek a homeostasis with our environment. The Van Orden Star reflects the state of balance we have struck, be it ideal or distorted. Any distortions of the apices of the Star reflect that individual's coming to terms with his personal space, his attempt to achieve balance.

Environmental constraints affect perceptual constancy and intersensory localization. Watch someone hitting a ball. If he sometimes hits, and sometimes misses, under the similar conditions, there is a lack of perceptual constancy, and intersensory localization. Temporal constraints manifest in postural shifts away from the vertical. For example, idiopathic scoliosis in teenagers is associated with a visual perceptual dysfunction, says Dr. Richard Herman, Orthopedic Surgeon, Good Samaritan Hospital, Phoenix, Arizona. When we observe shifts in posture, we can suspect they are functional, not structural. Many of us have observed this in traumatic brain injury patients. Some shuffle their feet, moving at a snail's pace; others walk on their toes, rushing along to maintain balance.The following figures represent the most frequently seen star patterns. You will see many variations, but these are representative of common presentations.

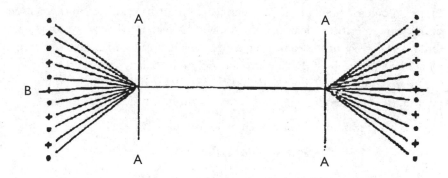

Figure A.7: Star pattern revealing optimal balance between temporal and spatial elements

Figure A.7 represents an optimal balance between temporal and spatial elements. The integrity of the illustration's planes and axes indicate a maximum balance in personal space.

Figure A.8 denotes constraints, in Macdonald's terms, of the peripheral-central relationship. My interpretation suggests that this pattern results when central demands supersede peripheral demands, and the individual selects a space location closer to him or her. The visible space world is rotated about the horizontal axis, bringing the sagittal plane closer, and directing the apices above the line. This type of individual will display behaviors associated with tunnel vision.

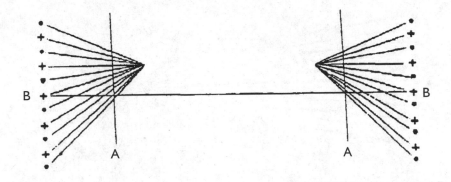

Figure A.8: Pattern caused by central demands superseding peripheral demands

Figure A.9 also represents constraints in the peripheral-central relationship. In this relationship, peripheral demands supersede focal. The visible space-world is again rotated about the horizontal axes, but here, the sagittal plane appears further away, and apices appear above the line. This pattern is usually associated with individuals who have increased near-point activity and visual stress.

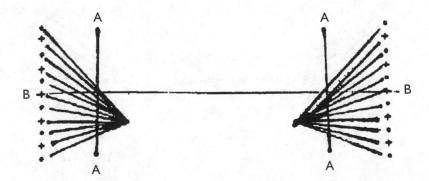

Figure A.9: Pattern caused by peripheral demands superseding focal demands

Figure A.10 displays constraints in the peripheral-central relationship that are manifested by disorganization of the visual system. The apices are poorly formed. Either they do not form an apex, as seen on the left side, or they form a fan shape, as seen on the right. These patients usually present a peripheral bias with no perceptual constancy. There may be an emotional component to the patients' visuo-spatial distortion.

In a study composed of 60 emotionally disturbed patients at the Westchester Medical Center and 60 control subjects, we compared far-point Van Orden Star

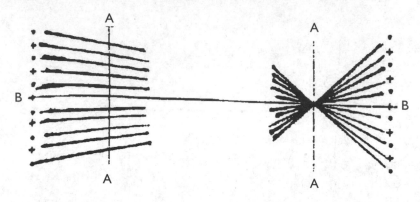

Figure A.10: Pattern showing disorganization of the visual system

patterns. There was a significant difference between the schizophrenic patients
and the control subjects. Typically, the schizophrenic subjects showed a crossing,
fan-like presentation on the right side, and no apex formation on the left
(P=0.003) (see Figure A.11). Compare this to a typical far-point drawing from
the control group (see Figure A.12).

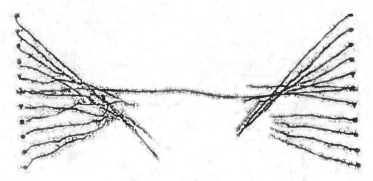

Figure A.11: Study showing far-point patterns in schizophrenic patients

Figure A.13 shows constraints in the peripheral-central relationship, which show
up as disorientation in the apices. These constraints are functional warps, and they
can be seen in physical performance as well as in a pencil-and-paper manifesta-
tion. For instance, when the patient is walking, a foot may toe in rather than point
straight ahead. The star pattern apices may be clearly formed, but they differ in
linear length. The pattern is rotated about the vertical axis, a projection of his or
her body image that is rotated around the mid-body axis. The subject's
perception of his or her space-world makes the frontal plane closer on the larger
apex side than on the shorter apex side.

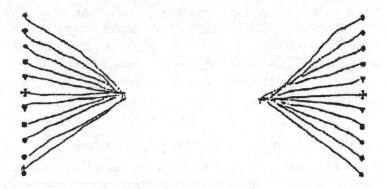

Figure A.12: Study showing far-point patterns in a control group

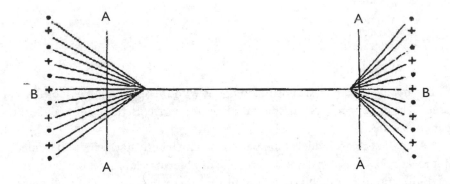

Figure A.13: Pattern showing disorientation in the apices

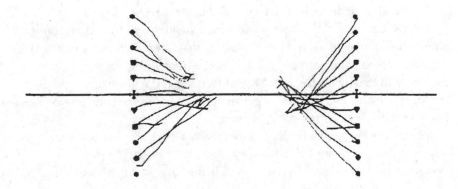

Figure A.14: Near-point testing pattern implying disorientation and disorganization

Figure A.14 represents constraints in the peripheral-central relationship that imply disorientation and disorganization. The Star has poorly formed apices. There is no apex on the left, and the right side forms a fan. There are many variations of this rendition, with apices being unequal along the frontal plane, or positioning above or below the midline. These star patterns are usually seen in individuals with concomitant visual and emotional issues.

Using the Van Orden Star to enhance your analysis

Clinical interpretation of the Van Orden Star can be a tool to recognize spatial behaviors. The spatially coordinated pattern is, fundamentally, a projection of the way behavior is molded and conditioned by temporal and environmental constraints. We know that visual thinking operates on a "what" and "where" system.

For an individual to interact with his or her environment, three questions must be answerable:

- Where am I?
- Where is it?
- What is it?

The temporal "where" system is homologous with the spatial ambient, or if you prefer, the peripheral, system: the star pattern can give useful insight about the patient's "where."

According to my model, a star pattern in which both apices are well formed, but meet below the line, depicts a problem of binocular coordination. This level of dysfunction has a relatively mild effect on the patient's sense of well-being. The pattern is commonly associated with near-point stress.

When the drawings end above the line but fail to meet in a definite apex, there is a more severe spatial organization problem. This pattern signals a temporal-spatial mismatch, and the individual's behavior will indicate a greater degree of stress.

As problems with the "where" system increase in severity, the digressions of pattern execution will increase. The key is that there is a mismatch in the magnitude of frontal plane design between the right and left fields. This represents an individual who has problems organizing the space-world, and at the same time is unable to orient self in personal space. It is not uncommon for these people to relate instances of panic behavior.

The concept of retinal rivalry has given way to a concept of cortical rivalry, with a division between the different aspects of the spatial system. A recent *Scientific American* article offered a tantalizing theory of where this is all happening in the brain.

In monkey studies during the late 1990's, only higher-cognitive areas—parts of the brain that process patterns and not raw sensory data—consistently fired in sync with changes in the animals' perception. That discovery buttressed a new theory: that the brain constructs conflicting representations of the scene, and that representations compete somehow for attention and consciousness.[5]

Now we can accept the fact that vision is not in the eye, but rather in the brain. When viewing the Van Orden Star, we see a representation of projected visual behaviors. The question that remains is: What do we do about it?

Lens application and the star pattern

For the past 25 years I have been a champion of yoked prisms, which I call ambient lenses, for the modification of human behavior. I have been prescribing them for individuals with learning differences, with emotional difficulties, and with autistic spectrum disorders. In addition, they have been very instrumental in rehabilitating traumatic brain injury cases.

In much of the literature on prism, it is the focal aspect of the lenses that is emphasized. Prism is prescribed in order to displace the image on the retina and align the foveae, producing single binocular vision. When an image enters a prism, it is compressed toward the prism base and expanded toward the apex. If prisms are applied in a yoked configuration, with binocular prisms oriented in the same direction, they induce spatial reorganization about the axes and planes of space. There is then a comparable shift in organization and orientation of the body, as directed by the incoming light.

Patients coming into my office are tested with the Van Orden Star and with Keystone Skills prior to coming into the examination room. These two tests give invaluable insight into the visual behavior of the patient. Often I can predict what findings will follow in the analytical, which in turn will confirm the preliminary findings.

The Van Orden Star supplies information as to the selective field, its organization and orientation. Behaviors can then be analyzed, and the type of lens needed for relearning selected.

Case in point, a 35-year-old adult male worked mainly at near point. He displayed the following information on the Keystone: exo posture near and far on the lateral muscle balance test, full fusion at far on the fusion test, but only 50 percent at near. The Van Orden Star had well-formed apices that met below the horizontal plane. As a result, I could predict that he was having trouble sustaining attention at work, had to reread to understand, and had problems maintaining his place when reading. The analytical showed poor positive fusional reserves at near, and high break and recovery of negative fusional reserves at near. All these indicated an application of yoked prism, base-up.

Clinical pearl: When apices are formed above the line, base-down prism is indicated. If apices are below the horizontal line, base-up is called for.

This interpretation of visual behavior from the star pattern, and the method of lens application, goes beyond the balance of central-peripheral function expressed by Van Orden, or the tight/loose organization described by MacDonald. I don't think it contradicts, but rather is an expansion of their thinking.

Prescribing of yoked prism, for me, started with a course of study at the Gesell Institute conducted by Dick Appel and John Streff. Streff introduced us to the work of Bruce Wolff, who had been using large-magnitude yoked prisms to alter behavior in his training room. I began using low-magnitude therapeutic lens prescriptions about 1972, and have written articles describing their use with learning-difference children.

Byall presented Figure A.15 and said, "This is (a common) pattern, and it indicates that the person is a 'straight-eyed squinter.'" (For all you non-dinosaurs, "squint" was the term commonly used for strabismus.) He would prescribe plus for the following reason: he felt that the frontal plane of the patient was postured too close, and was causing stress. Plus would allow the patient to posture further back in space, and gain relief. As I indicated earlier, to me this pattern reveals internal constraints that would interfere with spatial orientation, and the patient would physically exhibit a midline problem.

To cite another case: a 13-year-old girl from Massachusetts turned her foot in as she walked. She was having reading problems, and that was the reason for her coming to my office. Her Van Orden Star was similar to that of Figure A.13, but in

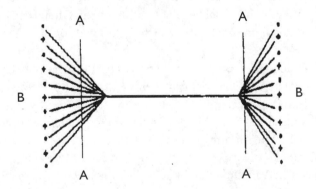

Figure A.15: Byall's pattern revealing internal constraints interfering with spatial orientation

her case the right apex was well formed but of greater magnitude than the left apex. I asked her mom, a nurse, "Would you like to see your daughter's feet point straight when she walks?" Her mother, with a quizzical look of disbelief, said, "Of course." I placed a pair of glasses on the girl with two base-right yoked prisms. When she started to walk with the glasses on, her toes pointed straight.

A similar case was that of a 75-year-old male stroke victim with unequal apices along the horizontal axis. His Van Orden pattern was more involved. His apices were disorganized. A dragging of his right foot marked his transport. With the use of yoked base-right prisms, his gait improved, as well as his balance. Both cases reported improvement when reading. Different degrees of constraint cause different levels of behavior difficulties. However, discrete lens application can raise any level of performance.

MacDonald's (1962–63) model of lens application was described by him thus:

> Prescribing lenses should be used to restore and maintain a balance of energies throughout the system. A plus lens will be used to flatten the input energy gradient, and reduce the energy input, into the system by spreading the energy over a greater area. A minus lens will tend to steepen the gradient and concentrate the energy … input into the system. As we view the system in operation, we should ask ourselves what effect the lens will have on the balance of the system.[6]

Clinical pearl: Base Up/Down for changes in organization
Base Left/Right for changes in orientation

Yoked prisms are one more tool we have to change the energy gradient in the patient's personal space. Prescribing base-up yoked prism rotates the visual level of attention to a lower, closer field of view. Yoked base-down prism rotates that level higher and further away. Both involve a rotation about the horizontal axis in space. There is a corresponding effect on the vergence system, improving spatial organization, sense of timing, and awareness of depth. Yoked base-right prism rotates the energy input about the vertical axis, moving attention toward the left field of view, while base-left moves it to the right. Laterally directed yoked prism affects the orientation of the body, and will influence the individual's posture, transport, and version eye movements.

Conclusions

Each of us has a personal way of viewing our environment. A tall person has a different view of his space-world than a short person. This can influence their posture and behavior. Our actions and reactions to our environment are orchestrated by temporal/spatial constraints.

When we perform an optometric examination, we are measuring an individual's adaptive response to his particular constraints. Wouldn't it be exciting to have a diagnostic tool that would give us insight into the personal space that governs our patients' performance? The Van Orden Star is just such a tool, and it can deliver the information quickly and accurately. The revealed patterns of visual behavior are reflections of behavioral patterns the patient has adopted. The paradigm presented gives an outline for the presentation, the interpretation, and the prescribing lenses from the Van Orden Star.

Notes

1   VO Star Patterns are available from Mast Development Co., Keystone View Division, 2212 E. 12th Street, Davenport, IA 52803, or Circle Publishing Co., P.O.Box 13073, St. Louis, MO 63110

2   Macdonald, L.W. 1962–63 "A Programmed Approach to Visual Training." *Visual Training 1*, 2, 9 and *Visual Training 1*, 5, 27.

3   Quick H.E. (1953) "Office Procedures for the Van Orden Star." *Visual Training at Work 7*, 39–42.

4   Byall R.S. (1955) "Interpretation of the Van Orden Star." *Visual Training at Work 4*, 8, 21–28.

5   Gibbs, W.W. (2001) "Side Splitting: Jokes, ice water and magnetism can change your view of the world – literally." *Scientific American*, January 18, 2001.

6   Macdonald, L.W. (1962–63) "A Programmed Approach to Visual Training." *Visual Training 1*, 2, 9 and *Visual Training 1*, 5, 27.

Glossary

AC/A RATIO: Accommodative convergence/accommodative ratio, measured in diopters. The degree to which the eyes turn inward in response to the amount of stimulus of accommodation (eye focusing).

ACCOMMODATION: The ability to focus upon targets at different distances, especially at near-point.

AFFERENT: Conveying inward toward a central location, as in nerves conducting signals to the brain.

AFFERENTATION: The conveying of impulses from the periphery to the central nervous system.

AMBIENT VISUAL PROCESSING: Vision of space. Often used synonymously with "transient" visual processing. Responsive to the low spatial frequencies (global information), can transmit discrete bits of information rapidly, and is thought to be involved in the perception of motion and depth, brightness discrimination, and the control of eye movements. Guides head and postural adjustments, and movement. Identifies the changing relationship between the body and spatial configurations of contours, surfaces, events and objects. Analogy: comparable to a wide angle lens, because it concentrates and miniaturizes a large field into a smaller framework.

AMBLYOPIA: The loss of central visual acuity that is not immediately correctable by the use of glasses or contact lenses. This may be the result of structural or functional defects, and may be either a developmental problem or an acquired problem due to trauma or head injury.

ANAGLYPH GLASSES: Glasses with one red and one green lens.

ANISOMETROPIA: Referring to an unequal balance in refractive status between the two eyes. It is not unusual to have a small refractive difference between the two eyes; however, this term is reserved for larger differences that may be detrimental to binocular perception and processing.

ANOMALOUS RETINAL CORRESPONDENCE: One of the adaptations that occurs in long-standing strabismus that allows for the foveal point of one eye to "connect" with a non-foveal point in the other eye in sending their simultaneous messages back to the occipital cortex.

197

ASTHENOPIA: Eyestrain (often accompanied by headache).

ASTIGMATISM: A refractive error causing blurred or distorted vision.

BINOCULAR VISION: The ability of both eyes to work together as a team. One result is stereopsis, or the ability to perceive three-dimensional space.

BODY SCHEMA: The knowledge of where one is in space, and where "self" ends and the outside world begins.

CONVERGENCE: Inward movement of the eyes in an effort to maintain binocular vision.

DEPTH PERCEPTION: The ability to judge the relative distance of objects.

DIOPTER: Unit used to measure the refractive power of a lens.

DIPLOPIA: Double vision.

ESOTROPIA: A type of strabismus where the visual system loses fusion and one eye turns inward toward the nose. Esotropia may be of developmental or acquired etiology.

EXOPHORIA: Under-focalization, repression of focal vision. The tendency for the eyes to aim at a point farther away from the patient than the object that is being focused upon. Exophoria does not involve a loss of fusion. It may be associated with headaches when visually concentrating, attention problems, and general visual discomfort. It is common in mild head injury patients, in whom it can cause attention deficits and an avoidance of reading and near-point tasks. Exophoria that occurs at the near-point is often referred to as a convergence insufficiency.

EXOTROPIA: A type of strabismus where the visual system loses fusion and one eye turns outward. Exotropia may be of developmental or acquired etiology.

FOCAL VISUAL PROCESSING: Vision of contour and objects. Often considered to be synonymous with "sustained" processing. Most sensitive to detail information, has a long response persistence. Figures are clear, while background blurs. It seems to be best designed for identification of color, form, shape and pattern resolution of fine detail. Comparable to a zoom lens magnifying a select area.

FOVEA: The portion of the retina where the finest detail vision (cone vision) is found. It is primarily concerned with sustained visual processing and is responsible for color vision.

FUSION: The simultaneous perception of visual input from the two eyes, forming a single perception of the surrounding visual environment. Fusion is lost when a misalignment of the visual axes occurs. It is necessary for proper development of binocularity.

HYPERCONVERGENCE: The mismatch that occurs when the eyes are aimed closer than the object being viewed.

HYPERMETROPIA: Farsightedness. See **hyperopia**.

HYPEROPIA: Also called "farsightedness." A condition in which light rays coming from a far object strike behind the retina. This is corrected with plus (convex) lenses.

HYPOCONVERGENCE: The mismatch that occurs when the eyes are aimed further than the object being viewed.

IDENTIFICATION: The labeling of the environment.

KINESTHETIC: A sensory experience mediated by nerve endings located in muscles, tendons and joints, which are stimulated by bodily movements and tensions.

"MINUS" LENSES: Conventional concave lenses prescribed for nearsightedness.

MYOPIA: Also called "nearsightedness." A condition in which light rays from a far object are brought into focus in front of the retina.

NYSTAGMUS: Involuntary side-to-side (or sometimes up-and-down) oscillations of the eye. Post-rotational nystagmus is a normal reflex that often is absent in autistic children.

OPHTHALMOSCOPE: A tool that allows an examiner to view the interior of the eye.

ORTHOPTICS: The diagnosis and treatment of ocular alignment problems through the use of non-surgical methods such as prism lenses and vision therapy.

PHORIA: A tendency for the eyes to be either vertically or horizontally misaligned.

PHOROMETRIC: Relating to measurement of phoria. See **phoria**.

"PLUS" LENSES: Convex lenses prescribed for farsightedness.

PRISM: A light transformer. A refracting medium that alters the direction (and subsequent localization) of light emanating from an object.

PROPRIOCEPTIVE SYSTEM: The sensory system that allows individuals to sense the position of their arms, legs and other body parts without seeing them.

PURSUITS: Tracking. The ability of the eyes to follow a slowly moving object without losses in fixation or associated jumpiness.

REFRACTIVE ERRORS: A clinical term used to describe the relative variation from emetropia (optimal) of the refractive power of the eye. Examples include hyperopia, myopia, and astigmatism.

RETINOSCOPE: An instrument used for objective measurement of refractive errors. The retinoscope is used to project light into the eye and then neutralize the movement of light reflection from the eye with lenses.

SACCADES: The ability of the two eyes to move from one point to another, while the visual information transmitted between these two points is suppressed. (These are also often referred to as fixations.) Uncoordinated eye tracking after trauma is often classified as saccades.

SAGITTAL: Pertaining to the imaginary plane dividing the body into right and left halves.

SCOLIOSIS: Lateral curvature of the spine.

SPATIAL ORGANIZATION: Awareness of the relationship between self and objects in all dimensions of the environment.

SPATIAL ORIENTATION: Awareness of the relationship between the body's axis and environmental positions.

STEREOPSIS: The ability of the eyes to discriminate small differences in depth when presented with alike yet disparate stimuli. It is one measure of two-eyed visual efficiency at the near-point and may also be referred to as third-degree fusion.

STIM: Self-stimulatory behavior, repetitive motor or vocal mannerisms to calm or excite the nervous system.

STRABISMUS: The collective term that refers to all binocular vision problems that involve a loss of fusion (i.e., exotropia, esotropia, hypertropia).

SUPPRESSION: The ability of the brain to "ignore" the visual input from one eye or the other. It is often an adaptive mechanism that develops as a result of strabismus, amblyopia or psychogenic disorders.

TACTILE: Pertaining to the sense of touch.

VESTIBULAR SYSTEM: The inner-ear system that helps us maintain our balance and informs us about our position in space.

VISUAL FIELD: The area of visibility when the eye is looking straight ahead.

Subject Index

Author Index